GOOD
MEDICINE

GOOD MEDICINE

The Art of Ethical Care in Canada

Philip C. Hébert, M.D.

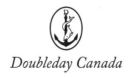

Doubleday Canada

Doubleday Canada and colophon are registered trademarks of Penguin Random House Canada Limited

Library and Archives Canada Cataloguing in Publication

Hébert, Philip C., author
Good medicine : the art of ethical care in Canada
/ Philip Hébert.

Issued in print and electronic formats.
ISBN 978-0-385-68325-8 (bound).—ISBN 978-0-385-68326-5 (epub)

1. Medical ethics.   I. Title.
R724.H394 2016   174.2   C2015-906227-6
C2015-906228-4

Book design: Kelly Hill
Cover images: J.D.S and Bariskina, both Shutterstock.com

Printed and bound in THE USA

Published in Canada by Doubleday Canada,
a division of Penguin Random House Canada Limited

www.penguinrandomhouse.ca

10 9 8 7 6 5 4 3 2 1

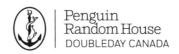

Penguin
Random House
DOUBLEDAY CANADA

This book is dedicated to Dr. Nathan Kaufman (1915–)
An extraordinary physician who knows the meaning of
surviving well and flourishing against all odds

"All changed, changed utterly."
W.B. YEATS, "Easter, 1916"

CONTENTS

Introduction: Strangers in a Strange Land   1

1   Bad Attitude   9

2   Plato and the Art of Letting Go   29

3   Thrown for a Loop   41

4   The Patient's Voice   65

5   A Death Foretold, a Death Unfolds   79

6   The Quality of Our Mercy   97

7   Suffer the Children   115

8   Quitting Time   135

9   Death and the Doctor   155

10   Beyond the Black Bag   173

Notes on Sources   185

Acknowledgements   191

Introduction

STRANGERS IN A STRANGE LAND

We all arrive as foreigners in the country of illness. Its flora and fauna, its language and customs are distinctive and challenging. The best guides for what can be a difficult and perplexing journey are knowledgeable and empathetic health care professionals. As there is almost always more than one path that patients might take, physicians, nurses, indeed all health care professionals must actively listen to patients and their loved ones so they can provide the best possible care. In turn, patients and their families must voice their concerns and openly share their stories so their health care professionals can understand how to best help them.

When it comes to serious illness, there is rarely an automatic passport allowing an easy entrance or exit. In modern medicine, the beginning or recognition of illness can be difficult. The end of illness can be complicated, too, and prolonged. The end is sometimes death, seen as a failure by many, as it sometimes is. But death may also come about through a process of consciously letting go. The challenge for all—health care providers, patients, and families—is to try to know when is the right time to do more and when is the time to let go. This book is partly about the process of letting go, but it is also about when we should *not* let go. It is about the experiences of patients and their families, and what we all should expect from a well-resourced health care system such as we have in Canada.

When Jane Mortimer was diagnosed with dementia in 2012, at the age of sixty-nine, she stated in what are known as advance instructions that she would not want "extraordinary measures" taken to keep her alive if she was unable to care for herself. Sadly, her dementia rapidly progressed, and she is now unable to speak or to feed herself. However, when offered food, she takes it, chews, and swallows. Despite Jane's written instructions, the nursing home where she resides refuses to stop feeding her, saying that feeding is not considered "extraordinary" care. Jane's family is unhappy with this situation and is uncertain what to do.

Gordie Howe—Mr. Hockey, one of the greatest hockey players of all time—was diagnosed with multi-infarct dementia (dementia caused by a series of strokes) at eighty-six years of age. Ravaged by his illness, he seemed lost, a shadow of his former self. He was virtually bedbound and had shed more than thirty pounds of his weight. His children, watching their father die little by little, in front of them, were unsure what to do. Gordie's neurologist said there was nothing more that could be done for him. Then an American company with a site in Mexico offered Gordie a novel and untested treatment with stem cell therapy. His family wasn't sure whether to accept it or not. The company had offered the therapy for free. "What have we got to lose?" one son argued. Gordie's neurologist was uncertain what to recommend. He had heard of such therapy but was worried about its dangers.

These scenarios are not uncommon in twenty-first-century medicine and will occur more and more frequently as our medical choices expand. In modern medicine we can almost always *do* things for patients. This is the era of medical miracles, after all. That does not mean we have a cure for some of the most serious diseases of the time, such as neurological illnesses like Huntington's, Parkinson's, multiple sclerosis, dementia, and brain cancer. But we can, with effort, imagination, and money, help some patients to some degree.

Before the twentieth century, patients had very little say over their care—"doctor's orders" held the day. Not that there was much for doctors to do—other than chopping off gangrenous limbs or pulling teeth or draining abscesses. Most medical care was ineffective, if not downright dangerous. "If the whole *material medica*, as now used, could be sunk to the bottom of the sea," observed Dr. Oliver Wendell Holmes in 1860, "it would be all the better for mankind—and all the worse for the fishes."[1] The well-known author and physician-administrator Lewis Thomas said of his own father, who was a doctor in the early years of the twentieth century, that his doctor's black bag carried only two useful things: morphine and magic.[2] (He added that patients were reassured just to see his father, and so he was, perhaps, his own strongest potion.)

Since then, science has radically and rapidly improved medical care. The black bag has become full of helpful drugs—and even more magic. By the mid-twentieth century, real choices became available to patients. Paired with the proliferation of medicine's scientific and technological advances were tremendous political and social shifts that caused medicine to tilt more positively in the patient's favour. It was as a result of the vigorous human rights movements in the 1950s and 1960s that the idea of choice—and patient autonomy—was fully recognized and came into rightful pre-eminence. The civil rights movement, the women's rights movement, the gay liberation movement, and the early AIDS movement, for example, all pushed medicine to adopt a more patient-oriented approach to decision making. Today there are alternatives of care that patients can consider, discuss, and choose between based on their own beliefs and desires. The idea of choice is a profoundly democratic one. It is bound up with notions of self-determination and privacy, and it represents an irresistible challenge to the authoritarian and paternalistic walls of traditional medicine.

Like many other professions, the medical profession has faced a loss of trust among the people it is meant to serve. This is, to some degree, a natural consequence of the evolution of medicine over the past century and the move away from its authoritarian roots. The nature of "good medicine" is changing, and this shift will leave some people happy and others dissatisfied. In my view, medical practitioners are responding to these challenges in largely positive ways. There is, for example, a deepened interest in understanding and preventing medical harm, and in basing treatment upon a critical understanding of what works and what does not. (Evidence-based medicine is a lot harder than you might think.) And beneath this is a constantly tested and renewed commitment among health care professionals to doing the best possible for their patients from the patient's point of view.

The new medical technologies, fuelled by research, have resulted in tremendous therapeutic improvements for the benefit of humankind. Yet one of the most powerful tools a doctor can employ is not technological but attitudinal: the skill of empathy. Empathy has been defined as the ability to enter into and inhabit the world of the other, which means, for medical professionals, the world of the patient. It means listening to the stories a patient tells, learning what life is like for the patient, and understanding what the patient thinks and feels and wishes about their medical care.

The ability to see the world through the eyes of another is a core ethical skill in medicine. True empathy cannot be faked. Patients and their families will sense if practitioners try to emulate it and do so insincerely.

Hence the important efforts—not to be discounted as just window dressing—during medical training to foster a type of medical care that best responds to and truly respects patients, their families, and their cultures. Medical trainees are now taught not solely anatomy and physiology but also how to care for the patient as a whole in their particular social circumstances—to treat patients as real people with concerns and issues that cannot always be resolved by science and technology alone.

This is the art of medicine, and while it has, at least since Hippocrates, always been taught in medicine, it is only in the past century that new tools of science, ethics, and law have allowed this art to be better appreciated and applied.

Lessons about empathy and the need for listening to patients' stories must be learned at the bedside and reinforced throughout a health care professional's training and practice, otherwise she or he may be overwhelmed by the everyday realities and constraints of medical care and the cynicism and despair these can induce. There are other important ethical values—of fairness, of respect, of compassion, of truthfulness, of sincerity, of integrity—that patients and families should also expect their health care practitioners to hold. Without them, things are apt to go less well for all involved, occasionally terribly so, and often in small but significant ways.

I entered the land of illness first as a physician and second as a patient. I trained as a family physician and was fortunate to be able to look after patients for more than twenty-five years. I have also been a patient for almost as many years. In the mid-1990s, when I was in my forties, I was diagnosed with Parkinson's disease. Between 2005 and 2009, I underwent six increasingly serious and debilitating surgeries for a series of back problems. I am still recovering from them. Ultimately, illness and disability forced my hand and, in 2010, I reluctantly retired from active practice, although not from medicine. Life rarely turns out as we envisage it.

Medical professionals are, more than ever, aware that they must have a humble and a critical attitude about what they think they know is "the best medicine." Medicine does not have all the answers, and accepted practice is often mistaken. To properly traverse this foreign land, patients must be heard, and their needs, desires, fears, and experiences reflected in how practitioners look after them. This book—the result of my experiences as a practising family doctor, as a medical ethicist, and as a patient with a serious illness—is about those necessary conversations, about the tragedy of voices not being heard, and the comfort that can be offered when they are.

To protect the privacy of patients, families, significant others, and health care practitioners, I have, except where noted, changed their names and altered some of their identifiable circumstances.

BAD ATTITUDE

"Doesn't sound good, does it, Doc?" Jerry Larson said to his family physician.

Jerry had been having problems for months before seeing Dr. Teeple. Food would get stuck in his throat when he swallowed. He tried to eat more slowly, carefully chewing every bite. But he had started choking on even small amounts of food. And swallowing began to hurt. When he weighed himself, he was startled to discover a fifteen-pound weight loss in just over two months. Then he began coughing up blood.

Jerry knew he should have gone to see Dr. Teeple then, but he kept putting it off. He had never been sick, didn't really know what it was to be sick, and didn't want to be sick. Finally, unable to ignore his symptoms any longer, he made the appointment.

The doctor asked Jerry how long he had been feeling ill. Was his swallowing becoming more difficult? More painful? Had he ever lost weight like this before? Did he have heartburn? Were his bowels normal? How bad was his coughing? Was his breathing affected?

Dr. Teeple examined Jerry briefly, listening to his chest and heart, and took his blood pressure. Then he shared some of his concerns. He wasn't exactly sure what was going on, he told Jerry, but he didn't like the possibilities. Dr. Teeple didn't say more. He didn't need to. Jerry knew his problem was serious.

Jerry was sent off for blood tests and a chest X-ray. Dr. Teeple's office called him two days later. The receptionist told Jerry that he was booked for an urgent appointment with a surgeon, Dr. Robert Caldwell, at a downtown teaching hospital. Jerry of course wanted to know more, but Dr. Teeple was out of the office and his receptionist did not have the authority to say why the referral had been made.

Jerry was one of the first patients I looked after as a fourth-year medical student during my two-month surgical rotation. It was 1983, and I was as green and uncertain as they come. However, as a clinical clerk, I typically had more time to spend with patients than the other members of the team. (I had even more time, actually, as I had broken my wrist at the start of the rotation, preventing me from attending at surgery.)

A widower for ten years, Jerry was a retired librarian and a book collector. He'd never been a father; books were his children, he said. He loved their smell, their binding, their texture, their scripts. Every book in his collection of four thousand or so volumes spoke to him. He hadn't read them all, but he could tell you when he had purchased or was given each one. Some people date their lives by music or their travels. Jerry did so by his book acquisitions.

I chatted with Jerry several times during his hospital stay. I was chastised by one clinician, who, impatient with my circuitous evaluation style, asked, "Are you interviewing the patient or having a conversation with him?" During my training, I had been taught that merely talking to patients was just not acceptable. I had learned to take a history from a patient in the most efficient, if impersonal, way. (This approach is not the only one or the best, as I would learn years later in my career. It left little room for hearing the patient's whole story or for developing an interest in and an understanding of the patient's values, unique history, and personality.)

As a student at the hospital where Dr. Caldwell practised, I had heard much about him. He almost always had a pipe in his mouth, and there were bets on whether he had ever lit it within the confines of the hospital. (He no doubt had, as, at that time, smoking was allowed anywhere in the hospital.) A general surgeon in a world of increasing specialization, he did bowel surgery, thoracic surgery, and bone and vascular operations. He had been at the hospital for decades.

Dr. Caldwell had been considered, at one time, a very good surgeon. But many felt he was past his prime. Rumour had it he was not very discriminating and would operate on almost anyone who appeared in his clinic. Around the time that Jerry went to see him, Dr. Caldwell seemed to have had a run of bad luck. His patients had experienced terrible post-operative complications, and a number had died in the intensive care unit. I don't think anyone thought to warn Jerry about this—certainly I didn't. I was a mere medical student, trying not to stray into anyone's firing range, attempting to be unobtrusive and not reveal my ignorance.

Jerry waited two hours to see Dr. Caldwell. The surgeon then hurried in and introduced himself, apologizing as he did so for keeping Jerry waiting. "Another emergency, sorry." Dr. Caldwell ushered him into his imposing office—always dark because he kept his blinds closed—and got right to the point. Chewing on his pipe, he pointed to some X-rays on a wall viewing box and said he had some bad news.

Jerry's X-ray showed he had a large mass in the central part of his chest. Jerry was told he would die unless it was cut out. Dr. Caldwell said he suspected an esophageal tumour, most likely malignant. To make certain, Jerry would need a scope examination, and a biopsy would have to be taken. As well, a CAT scan would enable the surgeon to see the extent of the tumour's spread.

Later, Jerry would tell me that at some point he stopped listening. He couldn't focus. All he noticed was, he said, the sweet smell of tobacco wafting from the surgeon's clothes. But his worst fears had been confirmed.

The endoscopy and biopsy confirmed that Jerry had squamous carcinoma of the esophagus. The CAT scan showed a large tumour extending from his upper stomach, invading adjoining structures, wrapping itself around major blood vessels, and reaching all the way to Jerry's heart. He would need surgery as soon as possible to remove the tumour.

"If you agree," Dr. Caldwell told him, "we'll take out what we can. Strip the tumour away from the vena cava and the heart." Later, Jerry could recall no in-depth discussions about the risks of surgery or his prognosis. "You are better off having surgery than not," he was told. Stunned, Jerry accepted the surgeon's recommendation and signed a consent form. He was too shocked to read the fine print. An OR spot was booked for the following week. Jerry was frightened of the operation, but the thought of a tumour growing unchecked in his chest was even more terrifying. He certainly didn't want to die.

"It doesn't seem like I have much choice," Jerry told me as I was admitting him to the surgery ward. "It's either have this operation or do nothing." Without the operation, he said, his esophagus would close off and he would choke on his own saliva. Not a pleasant way to die. Dr. Caldwell hoped the surgery would allow Jerry to swallow and give him a little more time.

I didn't—and couldn't, given my very limited experience—offer an opinion. But, having seen other poor patient outcomes on Dr. Caldwell's ward, I did not have a good feeling about the proposed operation. I felt powerless, as though I was watching an accident happen in slow motion.

Jerry's surgery was long and complicated.

When Dr. Caldwell visited Jerry in the recovery room, I tagged along. "We couldn't get it all, unfortunately," Dr. Caldwell told him. "We had to connect up what was left of your stomach to the part of your esophagus that we could salvage." *If you couldn't get it all, what was the point of the surgery?* Jerry wondered. *Now what?* Jerry felt too unwell at that moment to ask his surgeon these questions. When he expressed his disquiet to me later, I couldn't help but agree with him. *But what do I know?* I thought. *Nothing, really—nothing that could help Jerry.*

What Jerry did not anticipate was how ill he would be after surgery. Over the next two weeks, he seemed to get every post-operative complication in the book. His heart didn't function well and fluid backed up into his lungs, he had leakage from the operative site into his chest, he became septic from a hospital-acquired infection, and his kidneys started to fail. Then he had a stroke to the back of his brain, his vision centre, due to a septic embolism. Sudden blindness was the most disastrous complication for Jerry: he could no longer read. A quartet of friends sat by his bedside and read to him, but it was hardly the same as before.

On top of all this, Jerry had relentless pain—even to swallow fluids had become excruciating. "It's like swallowing glass," he told me. "What is the point of going on?" A feeding tube was inserted into his nose through to what was left of his stomach. This tube was even more painful for Jerry, so much so that he pulled it out. It was my job, as the junior member of the team, to make sure the feeding tube was properly placed.

"I'll do anything," Jerry pleaded, close to tears. "I'll try to drink fluids. Just don't put that tube down again!" But I was under orders from my resident to keep the tube in place. He didn't want the patient to die on his watch.

When I told the senior resident in surgery that Jerry objected to the feeding tube, he had but one response: "You want to let him starve to death?" I was told that I had a defeatist attitude. The idea, it seemed, was to do everything possible to prevent death. In this battle, what the patient wanted diminished to a vanishing point. Despite Jerry's objections, I reinserted his feeding tube time and again. Jerry didn't starve to death—he died two weeks later, with the hated feeding tube in place. Poor nutrition was the least of his worries. The causes of death included his cancer, his septic state, and his kidney failure.

I felt I had willingly but witlessly participated in an unnecessarily painful last rites ceremony. I had disobeyed that most basic axiom of medical ethics: "Above all, do no harm." I had ignored my patient's wishes concerning his treatment and so had abrogated my most fundamental professional responsibility: to provide the patient only with beneficial and desired treatment.

I did not know at the time that I could have declined to reinsert the tube or that Jerry had a right to refuse treatment. What are you supposed to do with a patient who appears to be choosing death over life? I knew almost nothing about the practicalities and realities of patients' rights or health providers' obligations. When I went through medical school in the early 1980s, we were never taught what to do if patients refused medical care. We did have a few dry lectures on medical law given by a lawyer, but they were very academic and hard to translate into clinical practice. Many students did not even bother to attend them.

But it is not just recognition of his legal rights that would have helped Jerry. I also didn't know that what is critical to good medical care is to understand what the patient wants and to begin from there. A better clinical sense would have spared Jerry some of his terrible suffering. In Jerry's case one could justify not tube feeding him on grounds of futility—he was going to die anyway, and no good would come from the tube feeding. He should not have had artificial feeding offered as anything more than, at best, palliative care, as comfort care, if he was hungry (which he was not). Things might have been different had there been real prospects that tube feeding would have improved his situation—but even then only if his decision making had been so impaired as to justify ignoring his wishes. That was not the case with Jerry. He was very ill and very unhappy, but, it seemed to me in my inexperienced way, he was quite capable of competently assessing what he was facing.

In our eagerness to keep Jerry alive, we had failed to comfort him.

Jerry's story is a relatively modern one, dating to the early 1980s, just before a seminal event in the history of medicine. In the 1990s two laws were passed in Ontario—one regarding consent to treatment and the other regarding substitute decision making. These laws express a fundamental but simple idea that health care treatment requires the true informed consent of a capable person. Patients must be able to understand their situation and the treatment alternatives available to them and must be able to choose freely among them. In cases where their decision making is impaired, patients have a right to have or name someone to be their "substitute decision maker." Jerry's case is evidence of why these laws were needed. These laws were meant to encourage conversation and communication between doctors and patients.

What Jerry lacked was an advocate. I didn't know how to play that role. It is now accepted that, except in emergencies, physicians generally cannot act as advocates for patients anyway. They cannot be "neutral patient-focused decision helpers" if they are the ones providing the intervention. The more risky and uncertain the intervention, the greater the need for an independent source of opinion. Family members (or friends who know the patient well) can and should play this role. But they, too, need to be informed and need to be prepared to ask difficult questions of the physicians. Jerry had no one in his corner and suffered as a result.

The ways I had failed Jerry have haunted me for years, and they fuelled my interest in medical ethics—the question of how medical practitioners *ought* to act towards their patients. That question, I was to learn, was an ethical one informed by an increasingly rigorous legal framework.

In 1980, the year I began medical school, the Supreme Court of Canada made a pivotal ruling on a case involving a forty-four-year-old Hamilton, Ontario, labourer, John Reibl, and his neurosurgeon, Dr. Robert Hughes.[1] In March 1970. Mr. Reibl consulted Dr. Hughes regarding his migraines. As part of his investigations, Dr. Hughes carried out an angiogram, to look at the blood circulation to Mr. Reibl's brain. He found that one of the main arteries was almost completely blocked by a clot. Although it was not causing Mr. Reibl any problems, and was not responsible for his migraines, Dr. Hughes recommended a carotid endarterectomy, a surgical procedure that removes the blockage by basically scraping out the clot. At the time it was all the fashion in medical practice. (It is now done less often and reserved largely for patients who have already had a small warning stroke triggered by a serious blockage in the circulation to the brain.)

Mr. Reibl agreed to have the procedure performed by Dr. Hughes. He would say later at trial that, while he knew there were some risks to the procedure, Dr. Hughes did not tell him what the exact risks were. Unfortunately, during the operation—which was conducted according to the technical standards of the day—part of a clot broke off, depriving a critical part of Mr. Reibl's brain of oxygen and causing permanent paralysis on one side of his body. Mr. Reibl was, as a consequence, unable to work.

Dr. Hughes had not warned Mr. Reibl of this complication, one that occurs in about one in seven cases. Thus, the procedure carried with it a not insignificant risk, even when performed by the best hands. Mr. Reibl was also unaware that there was no urgent need to remove the arterial blockage. Had he waited eighteen months to have the surgery, he would have been eligible for a full pension.

Mr. Reibl successfully sued Dr. Hughes for negligence in consent and was awarded compensation. The judgment was appealed, and eventually the Supreme Court ruled that any reasonable person, informed of the risks of the procedure and not in urgent need of the surgery, would have waited the eighteen months in order to be eligible for a full pension, just in case complications might occur. Dr. Hughes admitted that Mr. Reibl had asked him about the risks of paralysis resulting from the urgery. In responding to the question Dr. Hughes had emphasized that "the chances of him being paralyzed if he did not have the operation were greater than if he did have the operation." Dr. Hughes's defence had been, in part, that *most* doctors, perhaps not wanting to worry their patients, did not disclose the actual risks. The court was not impressed by this argument and concluded that a reasonable physician must tell patients what a reasonable person in the patient's position would need to know to make an informed choice.

Physicians needed to provide their patients with the information relevant to and necessary for true choice. Physicians needed to be "transparent." It was only in the 1980s that most North American clinicians had even begun to hear this message. A flurry of educational programs for physicians and other health care professionals were designed to help them understand just what the law now required. Many physicians at first decried this shift as the death of professionalism, but others saw it as the wave of the future—as a way of sharing decision making with patients and making the physician's burden of decision making less heavy.

But many questions remained. How much information was enough to obtain valid consent from a patient? Should the standard be how much other doctors told their patients? Should the standard be what a "reasonable person" would need to know to make a "reasonable decision"? Or should doctors be expected to know, and tailor their disclosure to, every patient's individual situation and beliefs? Until the case of Mr. Reibl, it was not clear what the standard should be for physicians. How could we expect a doctor to know about a patient's *pension eligibility*?

The answer is that Dr. Hughes need not have known about that. But his patient needed to be warned by the doctor of the risks and complications that might occur with *and* without surgery, so he could evaluate for himself his options and their potential risks. Had Dr. Hughes fully informed his patient, it is the *patient* who would have borne the responsibility for the outcomes of his choice.

The role and limits of transparency in disclosure were further refined in 1997, in the case of Carole Arndt. Here, to the surprise of some, the Supreme Court ruled that the doctor's failure to be transparent was *not* found to be negligent.[2] In the 1980s, Ms. Arndt had had a hard time getting and remaining pregnant. She and her spouse were both skeptical of mainstream medicine. When she did get pregnant, in 1986, the couple booked a midwife for her delivery. But during the twelfth week of this much-wanted pregnancy, Ms. Arndt came down with chicken pox, an infection she had not had as a child. She went to see her family doctor, Dr. Smith, concerned about the effects exposure to the virus might have on her fetus.

Uncertain of the answer, Dr. Smith spent part of the next weekend in the library. She wanted to provide accurate information to Ms. Arndt and her husband, without causing them undue worry. What she discovered was that only 2 per cent of babies exposed to the varicella virus before birth will have birth defects. Of these, fewer than one in five hundred would have serious brain and motor problems, and some of those would die early in life. Dr. Smith decided not to warn Ms. Arndt and her husband, because these terrifying prospects struck her as too remote and so not a good reason to prematurely terminate a hard-to-achieve pregnancy. Unfortunately, Ms. Arndt's daughter, Miranda, was born with the most serious form of what is known as congenital varicella syndrome. She had, among other problems, marked neurological under-development causing her severe cognitive impairment and serious intestinal problems that required tube feeding. Over the next eight years, she had undergone a number of surgeries and would need life-long institutional care, a life that would be shortened by her condition.

Miranda's parents sued Dr. Smith. They said at the trial that, if Dr. Smith had properly informed them (as a reasonable doctor would have) of the more serious risks of varicella exposure to the fetus, they would have opted to terminate the pregnancy. Not being properly cautioned by their doctor, they argued, deprived them of a choice that should have been theirs to make.

The lawyer representing Ms. Arndt asked Dr. Smith, "You in fact knew when you told me that you indeed hadn't told her what you had learned, isn't that correct?"

"I hadn't told her all that I had learned," Dr. Smith replied.

"You hadn't told her of—of the most serious defects that you had learned about, isn't that correct?"

"I didn't tell her about the cortical atrophy, the mental retardation and so on, no."

"You only told her about skin and muscle problems?"

"Yes. Those were reported as the most frequent."

"You didn't tell her about those risks that could be most harmful to the fetus, isn't that correct?"

Dr. Smith agreed. "Yes, I didn't tell her."

For the trial judge, Dr. Smith's failure to disclose to Ms. Arndt all the serious risks amounted to medical negligence. The doctor had deliberately not warned Ms. Arndt and her husband of the serious risks because *she* thought the risk to the fetus was very small and not a reason to warrant an abortion. She thus took unto herself a decision that should have been made by the parents.

So, this should have been a straightforward decision: the doctor had a duty of care to the parents, she failed to meet the standard of care (of disclosure) to the parents, and an injury occurred to them (the birth of a child with severe deformities). However, the court did not find the cause of the injury was the failure of the doctor to disclose the risk, as it felt the parents, given their beliefs, would not have chosen an abortion even if they had been fully apprised of the risks. These findings were appealed to the Supreme Court of Canada.

The Supreme Court agreed, in 1997, that Dr. Smith did *not* disclose what a reasonable patient (the parents) would want to know. However, the majority decided that for *these* parents, *this* reasonable expectation of full disclosure's not being met would have made no difference to their decision to have the child. And if the information would make *no* difference to the patient's decision, then it is not necessary to share it, and there can be no negligence in its non-disclosure. The court reasoned that, because Ms. Arndt had a "suspicion of the mainstream medical profession," even if she had been properly warned, she would not have opted for an abortion. Hence, the Supreme Court ruled, Ms. Arndt and her husband could not claim an injury. The legal test for disclosure was not one of *total* transparency; rather, it rested on disclosing the information to the patient that would make a difference to his or her decision making.

When things do not go as expected and patients sue doctors for failure to obtain an adequate consent (what is called "negligent consent"), the courts, in eight out of ten cases, decide *against* the patient.[3] This may be because the courts often think, as in this case, that the patient would have made the *same* decision about the procedure even if their doctor had warned them of the risk beforehand.

If Ms. Arndt and her spouse had been adherents of mainstream medicine, then the doctor would likely have been found negligent. Perhaps Dr. Smith knew her patients well enough to know that they would not act on the information she had discovered. Or maybe the doctor was just lucky.

Was Jerry given all the information he needed to make a reasonable decision? Did he know how desperate a manoeuvre his surgery was—and that there was no chance of cure? Was he aware of how terrible the outcomes of his type of invasive procedure could be? Or of the outcomes suffered by other patients? If not, his consent to the surgery was not valid in the first place. Although Jerry was gravely ill after his surgery, I don't think anyone ever sat with him to tell him that he was dying and that his options were limited. It is this compassionate communication, a simple, if hard-to-begin, conversation, based on an empathetic appreciation of Jerry's situation, that could have eased his suffering better than any technical intervention at that point.

Of course doctors are never sued for providing too much information, only for providing too little. More information can help most people. It would not likely have helped extend Jerry's life. It might, however, have made his last few weeks or months more tolerable. Perhaps if he had been told how bad things were for him, he might have opted for palliative care rather than surgery. Other options, such as dilating the esophagus or radiating the tumour, might have been explored as well. None of these would likely have extended his life, but the quality of his life might have been better. The narrative of his life had an ending that was harsh and cruel; it could have ended better, if he had written his own ending, rather than having it written for him. It bothers me still that I knew what Jerry wanted and acted against his wishes.

In Jerry's case there was also the question of whether Dr. Caldwell's recent surgical record would have influenced his decision to consent to the surgery. A spate of deaths among children who had had heart surgery in Winnipeg in the mid-1990s resulted in a public inquiry led by Justice Murray Sinclair.[4] One of the recommendations coming out of this inquiry was that physicians, in obtaining consent for a surgical procedure, should disclose not just the profession-wide risks of the procedure but also, and perhaps more importantly, the risks of the procedure if done in *that* particular hospital or by *that* particular physician. The relevance of such information to patient and family decision making is obvious.

The fact is that medical trainees *can* learn and *are* now learning how to better listen to patients. Medical students in Canada and the United States are now being taught the lessons inherent in these stories, and are learning as well the skills needed to best respect patients' views and preferences. These skills are not difficult to learn, although practice and experience make doctors much better at it.

These are also hardly new subjects in medical schools, but there is a new and increased emphasis on them. "Professionalism," it is rightly called—learning the conduct becoming a physician—and it is, thankfully, transforming medical education everywhere and, as a result, also, slowly, changing medical professionals everywhere.

The hospital where I trained, and where Jerry died, has since been demolished. What happened to Jerry—that he was not listened to and had no control over his dying process—should be a thing of the past, too.

II

PLATO AND THE
ART OF LETTING GO

Plato was doing his best to die on me. I didn't want him to die and didn't think he needed to die. I was his primary care M.D. *There is no reason for him to die*, I thought. *No good reason, anyway.* But Plato (in this case his *real* name) was a stubborn man.

Plato and his wife, Irene, had been my patients for almost two years. Not long after I had finished my residency program in family medicine, I had joined a community clinic and taken over their care from a retiring physician who had known them for years. Plato's visits to the clinic were welcomed by all the staff. He was not a complainer; he was low maintenance, as we say in the medical business. Plato had, in my estimation (and in his, too), a good quality of life. He was a retired architect of some renown. He was well read and kept up on current events. He was also easy to like—always ready with a smile, always a bounce in his step. He would come to the clinic wearing a blue serge suit or a herringbone jacket and sporting a bow tie, looking like he was ready for a day at the office. Irene, willowy and glamorous, was also always well turned out, in pearls and slim dresses, the better to show off her trim physique. In the 1930s she had danced with a Russian ballet troupe. Now in her eighties, she liked to show me how flexible she still was, how easily she could still touch her toes. I envied her suppleness.

The two had been together a long time, married for fifty-five years. Irene left Stalin's Russia for France in the late 1930s. Plato had fought in the Greek resistance under the leadership of Aris Velouchiotis. The failure of the rebellion forced him into exile in France, where he and Irene met in the last days of WWII. Starving and grieving the loss of many family members, they escaped together from the ruins of Europe to Canada.

Visiting a doctor was a special occasion for Plato and Irene. Plato listened carefully and respectfully to what the doctors (and nurses) told him. Irene was more forward, and would question our recommendations, but beneath that veneer of suspiciousness was simply someone who cared deeply about her spouse and was going to make sure he (as well as she) received the best possible care. Although part of a respectful generation, she felt comfortable challenging their care providers if she felt she was not listened to or not taken seriously.

I was almost as stunned as Plato was by Irene's sudden death. While she was out shopping one day, she had an arrhythmia, or a change in the normal heartbeat, and dropped dead. Plato was devastated. Afterwards, he looked at me so intensely that I wondered if he thought I had missed something in caring for Irene. *If I had been more vigilant, perhaps she would still be alive. Maybe.* I left my thoughts unsaid.

After Irene's death, Plato, too, developed a heart problem. He was in and out of the ER and hospital four times in twelve months with congestive heart failure. Known as CHF for short, it has many causes—heart attacks, diseased heart valves, kidney problems, drugs— but the common result is the heart's inability to pump blood as it should. Patients become unable to breathe as fluid backs up into their lungs and often into their liver and legs. They literally drown in their own fluids. With each episode, the resilience of Plato's heart and lungs would be diminished just a little more, his heart more soggy, his lungs more resistant to shunting oxygen.

Now Plato was back in the ER for a *fifth* time. He allowed himself—reluctantly—to be brought in by ambulance when a neighbour noticed he didn't look so well and he was having trouble breathing. He didn't want to come to hospital. Plato thought that the emergency room had more important patients to attend to than himself.

His condition, with treatment, improved. Soon he was able to breathe better, and the heaviness in his chest lifted. The cardiologist who had been consulted wanted to keep him in hospital. "If he goes home now," said the cardiologist to me when I later arrived in the ER, "he'll just be back next week." There was a note of cynicism in his voice, as if he had seen this all before, as if Plato was there for the attention and coddling. Plato had told the hospital staff that he wanted to go home, but they weren't paying much attention to his protestations. They assumed that he wanted to stay.

I had gone to the ER after Plato's situation was brought to my attention by our community nurse, Mary Ann Carter. Mary Ann worked in the community clinic with me. She was the real go-between for patients and doctors. (The termination of her position after this story took place was a terrible setback for keeping patients' interests at the fore of the clinic's mission.) Mary Ann told me that Plato wanted us to help him get back home.

Mary Ann and I visited Plato in the ER. We asked him how he was doing.

"I've had enough," he said. "I'm through with life."

It was unlike Plato to be so bleak, and it shook me. Plato was the first patient of mine to decline life-sustaining care. I had yet to receive much guidance about how to handle a situation like this.

At eighty-eight, Plato had survived a tremendous amount of change in his lifetime, but, he said, he had lost interest in life since Irene's death. He told us that it was as if he had been wandering in a desert, parched, ever since Irene had died.

Plato and Irene had a son, but Plato said he was a "no-goodnik" who could not be relied on for anything. "He's got his own life," Plato said to me. "Don't bother him." There was a note of resignation, more than bitterness or blame, in his voice. In the decade or so that Plato and his wife had been coming to the clinic, their son had been seen only two or three times. One of those times was to get a medical certificate to attest to Plato's mental capacity to change his will, leaving more of their estate to him.

Now Plato felt his own death was near; he welcomed it, and his only fear was dying in hospital. "It's the worst fate," Plato said to us, "that a man should die in hospital."

In Greece the elderly were taken home by their family and cared for until they died. But without Irene, Plato had no family to help him. He had outlived all his friends. He'd gotten so old, he said, that even some of the buildings he'd designed decades ago were being torn down and replaced by condos. "What is the point of going on?" he asked Mary Ann and me. He felt he had outlived his time. I wondered if he was right.

Nowadays, when physicians are uncertain about what to do, we gather information beyond the purely medical. What does the patient want, and why? What is life like for the patient? Nowadays, doctors are taught to listen to their patients, to use a radar-like sensitivity to understand their patients' lives, to engage them in critical conversations. But in 1989, when Plato confronted me with his desire to die, it was something I had yet to fully understand.

Plato just wanted to be left alone, in his own home, to die. I believed he was asking us to provide him with less than optimal care. I knew what CHF was, what caused it, and how to treat it (with diuretics, digoxin, ACE inhibitors, etc.). If my knowledge as a family doctor was stretched as regards treating CHF, I could always consult my favourite cardiologist about what to do. This is what physicians were taught: provide the best medical care, improving the patient's quality of life and extending it where possible.

But in Plato's case it was not a question of *how* to do something but rather of *what* to do—and *whether* to do anything at all. In these circumstances, a medical specialist is unlikely to know better than a generalist what to do. In fact, if the best treatment is the one most consistent with the patient's values and wishes, the generalist or family doctor may be in a better position to know what the patient would want.

Doctors must know not just how but *when* to use their expertise—when to press onward and when to pull back. Plato was mentally competent. Going home to die was what he truly wanted and expected. He told me that when he got home, he would stop taking his pills and die. He wanted my help in making his death peaceful.

Was Plato's refusal of care so undeniably unacceptable, so despairing, that it should not have even been entertained by his doctors and nurses?

It is possible to underestimate the resilience of patients with depression if you are captured in their orbit of despair. Given some effort and imagination, we might have been able to identify and modify various factors influencing Plato's wish to die—the rift with his son, his isolation, his sad and failing heart.

From *my* perspective, anyway, Plato had a lot to live for. I enjoyed his company, his stories, his "being-in-the-world." I wished Plato had had a more helpful, support-ive family—someone to look after him, to care for him. I couldn't help but think that, were he not so alone, his despair would not have been so deep, and his desire to die not so intransigent.

Mary Anne had known Plato much longer than I. She was reluctant to let him go home alone. She would fol-low him home when he did go. She was afraid about what might happen to him if she were not around. I, too, was concerned. I made house calls, but I could not be there all the time.

Mary Ann and I decided to help Plato go home, but I needed to be sure of a few things first.

"How do you know you won't panic when your breathing worsens?" I asked him. "The cardiologist says it *will* get worse. He's probably right. There is only so much I can do for you at home."

"Just do the best you can," he replied, looking away from me. "That cardiologist is a worrywart. I'm so tired here. I can't sleep. It's so noisy and at night the nurses come in every two hours to make sure I haven't died yet."

"It's just for that reason everyone thinks you should stay in hospital—well, everyone except Mary Ann, that is. She thinks you have a right to go home, just not alone. She's pretty skeptical that we can do much for you in the long run."

"Well, Doctor, what do *you* think? I know I don't want to stay here."

"I don't know what to recommend, Plato. I hear you when you say you want to get out of here, but I'm afraid that you'll be at home all alone and you'll get worse again. Look, maybe you're depressed. Would you agree to see a psychiatrist here, a very nice one who has strong views about not abandoning the elderly? Maybe she could help."

"No, I don't think so, but thank you, Doctor."

"What about help at home—maybe live-in help? You could afford it."

"Again, thanks, but no thanks. I just need you and Mary Ann. I don't want strangers in my house."

As a last resort, I decided, with some guilt in my gut, to use the only trump card I had left. "What about *Irene*? What do you think she would want you to do?"

Plato didn't hesitate. "She'd want me to do whatever I felt I needed to do. But only after she had called me a stupid ass, of course." Plato smiled.

I had to laugh. His spark was still there. I could imagine her saying exactly that with a gleam in her eye.

We couldn't keep him in hospital, tied down. For Plato there was no light at the end of the tunnel.

When Plato got home, he did as he had promised— he stopped taking his pills, and soon stopped eating as well. He would only take sips of ice water. Mary Ann and I met at his house. It was filled with art and Lalique crystal. *What a beautiful place to die*, I thought.

Plato offered me a piece of the crystal, but I couldn't accept it. We talked a little about the city and architecture, about Irene. But, given his frail state, he did not remain lucid for long. He lapsed into a delirium and died at home in less than a week. His son never appeared.

Mary Ann was there at the end. She told me Plato's death was peaceful. Mary Ann, though sad, was sure we had done the right thing by him. She had no doubts about this.

I have often thought about Plato and Irene since. Should I have been more vigilant with Irene? Should I have been more forceful about Plato's care? Did I too quickly concur with his decision to leave hospital against medical advice? Did we too readily agree to Plato's wish for a quick exit because he was an old guy? What if he had been thirty or forty years younger? What would have been "reasonable" then?

Ultimately, it is the patient who must decide whether or not to accept treatment. This is the fundamental lesson I learned from Plato. But things are never so simple as that. How much effort did we really put into addressing the issues that might have made a difference for Plato? It seems so much easier to allow someone to refuse care than to seek the changes in their social and emotional environment that would support them and help them thrive, not just survive. This is a failing that sometimes doctors and nurses feel as a sense of helplessness. But it was—and still is—reflective of a failure in how we, as a society, provide care. People are seen for intermittent episodes of illness. We do not follow them after the late-night ER visits. Nor do we provide them with any comprehensive follow-up or loving care.

The social determinants of illness cannot be treated with the same precision and skill as the more direct biological causes of illness. Doctors and nurses are not social engineers. Medicine on its own cannot solve all the problems it encounters. Knowing just when is the right time to let a patient go requires years to learn. Patients often know long before doctors do, and it is a skilled clinician who knows how to listen to and accommodate a patient who wants to let go. I did not have the years of experience when Plato was in the hospital to be sure we were doing the right thing. I very much relied upon Mary Ann's experience and street smarts. Could we have done something differently? Perhaps we could have arranged a home visit by a geriatric specialist. We might have more strongly encouraged the use of antidepressant treatment. Perhaps a home visitors program. Maybe a more determined effort to contact his estranged son. In the end, however, I do not believe that any of this would have helped. Plato was too anxious to be done with life. It would have been like rearranging the deck chairs on a sinking *Titanic*.

Time has eased my regrets about Plato and Irene, but it has not erased them. That is probably how it should be. Letting go of the thread of a patient's life should be neither rushed nor easy. I learned early on in my training that not all patients can or even ought to be saved. How we do, and should, respond to critical illness can be a fragile undertaking, fraught with uncertainty. Whether as a patient, a family member, or a health care professional in the midst of the crisis of an illness, no one is free of regrets. Everyone thinks, *If only circumstances had been different.*

It is difficult to pass the thread of a patient's life through the eye of the needle of good, reasonable medical care. This can be, at times, a seemingly impossible task. There are so many uncertainties and complexities; it is so hard to get it right and all too easy to get it wrong. We sometimes let the threads of life go when we ought not to. At other times we try to keep stitching a life together even though it is disintegrating before us. That does not mean we shouldn't try to get it right. Or at least try to do it better.

The treatment that a patient chooses can turn out in ways that are neither expected nor desired. The result may be one that is complex and unforeseen by all. I know this more deeply now having been a patient myself for many years and traversed the country of illness.

III

THROWN FOR A LOOP

The worst thing about brain surgery, if you're awake, is when they drill through your skull.

It was the summer of 2014, and my surgeon was drilling two quarter-sized holes *in my head*—one on each side, close to my receding hairline. It sounded as if I was standing next to a 747 jet engine, and the reverberations felt as though someone was taking a jackhammer to my head. I was also aware of the sickening acrid smell of burning bone—*my bone*. My instinct was to leap off the table, but I was locked in place.

My God, what have I got myself into?

Yes, my walking had become worse, but would this surgery really be the solution? My skull seemed altogether too thick at that point. As the drilling continued, I became very tearful, on the verge of losing my composure.

I was shaking like a leaf. I had the silly thought that I, being a doctor, should understand the surgical process and so be immune to any emotion. But I was not immune and I couldn't stop asking: *What am I doing here?* I was semiprone, my head immobilzed by a steel frame, and the neurosurgical team positioned largely behind me and out of view. I could see my surgeon, Dr. Misra; he was to one side, directing the larger surgical team like a conductor. I hoped he wouldn't notice how upset I was. I prayed his team knew what they were doing.

Then, suddenly, the nurse anaesthetist was there, holding my hand. "It will all be okay," she said in a calm and soothing voice. "Everyone gets nervous. Hang on." I would rely on her tranquility more than once over the next five hours. Just her being there was reassuring. I felt less alone.

Having brain surgery turned out to be the best decision I have ever made. It was to be life-transforming for me in the most positive of ways. It would give me my life back.

I have had Parkinson's disease for more than twenty years. Parkinson's is what we call a neurodegenerative illness, meaning it results in loss of nerve function. Its cause is unknown and its severity is variable. It almost always worsens with time: everything slows down, movement becomes difficult, and cognitive impairment occurs in many patients.

For more than a century, surgery has been considered an accepted treatment for Parkinson's. In the late 1800s it was observed that Parkinson's patients who suffered strokes or had lesions in certain areas of their brains might experience a dramatic improvement in their symptoms—the shaking, the stiffness, the walking abnormalities that characterize Parkinson's. No one knew why, but it led doctors in the 1920s to remove those parts of the brain apparently responsible for the symptoms of Parkinson's.

Then, in the 1960s and 1970s, the discovery that it was a deficiency of the neurochemical dopamine that caused Parkinson's revolutionized treatment. Dramatic changes in patients with severe Parkinson's were seen when they received L-dopa, the medicinal formulation of dopamine.[1] Brain surgery suddenly seemed outmoded, bypassed as a dangerous exercise of surgical excess. The initial and standard treatment became, and remains, dopamine replacement by way of various medications.

But in the past decade, advances in surgery—less risky, less invasive forms of surgery—have begun to change the calculus of benefits and burdens attending to decisions about Parkinson's treatment. Deep brain stimulation, or DBS, was one of these new surgical options and a relatively low-risk one. DBS has been performed on tens of thousands of patients worldwide. (Still, by all accounts it is considered appropriate and most helpful for only about 15 per cent of Parkinson's patients.)

I knew about DBS—vaguely, anyway—but for years I had no interest in pursuing any type of surgery for my Parkinson's. It seemed too frightening, too irreversible an option. Whenever you open the brain, there are small but serious risks: infection, stroke, bleeding, and personality changes—patients can become impulsive, depressed, even lose some of their cognitive capacities, their ability to think and to be themselves. I felt that I wasn't "bad enough" to need any type of surgery. *This is my brain—it's where I live*, I thought. *What if they screw it up?* On top of that, between 2005 and 2009, I underwent a number of less than successful and increasingly gruesome back operations that had made me extremely risk-averse about surgery.

However, my neurologist, Dr. Shelly Duncan, kept mentioning that I would be a good candidate for several types of surgery for my Parkinson's. She meant that I was relatively young, otherwise well, and still responded to dopamine, although its efficacy for me was clearly waning. I was experiencing longer periods of stiffness, and my ability to walk, in particular, was declining. For more than a year, just crossing the street had become arduous, leaving me exhausted and sweating profusely. My self-confidence and optimism were dropping like dead weights in the water. And so I decided to put myself in the hands of surgeons. I opted for DBS, one of the newer surgical options. I was somewhat reassured that nothing would be removed from my brain; only very thin wires would be threaded into it.

Although my neurologist was sure the operation would help me, that I was a good candidate, I delayed making my decision. I was unconvinced. Part of my initial panic about the operation was my lingering worry that I did not, in fact, even have Parkinson's. I wondered if I had not rushed too fast into having my skull pried open.

That's how much denial I harboured.

My neurological problems had started simply enough in the 1980s, when I was in my mid-thirties and, having finished a residency in family medicine, I was working in a small town in northern Ontario. (At the age of twenty-nine, I had come to medicine much later than most of my classmates. I had spent ten years in the 1970s as a student of philosophy before medical school.) Gradually, insidiously, my left foot and ankle started to feel odd. My foot would turn inwards and cramp up. At the time I thought that I was running too much or maybe I was running too infrequently. Was it arthritis, a mechanical problem, my circulation, maybe? I tried fancy orthotics, new shoes, various foot braces and elaborate exercises. I even took dance classes. Nothing worked.

I had never considered myself a hypochondriac. Now I wondered if I was becoming one. I was starting to understand what patients experience when they have unexplained symptoms. I had to sort this out, and so I had a brain scan done. The results were normal. I kept hobbling along for another two years.

In late 1994, I saw Dr. Michael Orlov, a neurologist at a teaching hospital in Toronto. Dr. Orlov was a specialist in multiple sclerosis, one of the few in the city. I wasn't expecting any great revelations, so I didn't ask my wife, also a physician, to come along with me. I didn't think I had MS and I knew I had not had a stroke. Dr. Orlov listened to my story, examined me with care, looked over my test results.

"You don't have MS, I'm sure of that," he said. Then, out of the blue: "What about Parkinson's disease? Has anyone considered that?"

"No," I said. "No one has ever mentioned it as a possibility."

I believed in being honest with patients, but Dr. Orlov's question was a bit blunt. Still, it was a possibility that could not be sugar-coated.

My mind flashed to two of my elderly patients with Parkinson's in the chronic care wing of my hospital. One, a retired doctor, had marked cognitive impairment and would walk around the halls naked. "I'm just an old goof," he would say, his medical career long forgotten. The other patient, like an untethered windmill, suffered from dramatic, involuntary writhing motions in his limbs (a condition known as choreoathetosis), perhaps due to the high doses of dopamine he had been taking for so long. I was used to diagnosing Parkinson's in my elderly patients. Now *I* was the patient.

"But I'm only in my thirties. I thought only old guys got this disease!"

"In fact 10 per cent of Parkinson's patients are under fifty years of age when they are diagnosed," Dr. Orlov replied.

I felt as if I was falling backwards into someone else's life. Was it really *me* he was talking about? How was I to take it? How would I cope? How long would I last?

"But I can't have Parkinson's. My second child will be born soon. How can I be a father to him? And what about my work as a doctor? How will I be five years from now?" I didn't want to even think about ten or twenty years down the road.

Dr. Orlov said that he couldn't predict the future. Some people decline quickly, he said, others less so. He was realistic. "There are good desk jobs in medicine," he assured me. But I wanted to look after patients, not be a paper-pusher.

"Will I ever be able to run again?" I recalled racing through the countryside, long before my illness.

"Don't count on it," Dr. Orlov replied, shrugging. "In any case," he said, "you should try dopamine replacement. If it helps you, then you almost certainly have Parkinson's." I should have felt anger or frustration, but I couldn't summon up these feelings. I think I was in shock. I left the neurologist's office, clutching my prescription, experiencing a kind of relief and also a certain terror. True, I had an explanation for my ailments. My condition was serious and not imaginary. And I had a drug that might help me. As well, I guess I was happy not to have MS. But otherwise the advantages of the diagnosis seemed few.

My wife was as taken aback as I was by the news. "Are they sure? You don't look like a Parkinson's patient." I had to agree. But I had no better explanation. Over the next year I would seek the opinions of other neurologists; they all concurred with Dr. Orlov.

I started on dopamine replacement therapy and, although I did not feel myself again, my walking was a little better, my balance was enhanced, and my penmanship improved. The real proof of my improvement came from an unexpected source. Within a week I received a small plaque from the nurses on the chronic care ward where I worked. It was for the "most improved handwriting of any doctor on the ward." I laughed at this *(If they only knew . . .)*, and considered it prophetic: my diagnosis was truly affirmed.

At first, only my wife and children knew that I had Parkinson's. It was two years before I told even a few close friends. They deserved, I thought, an explanation for why I was limping about. It was three or four years before I felt I could tell my siblings, even longer before I told my colleagues, and, last of all, after eight or nine years, my patients.

But before I could tell my patients about my Parkinson's, there was a bright summer day in 2002. We were on Toronto Island with our young children. I was still walking with difficulty but, when I noticed a group of people racing on the lake, I thought to myself, *I can do that.* So I joined a competitive rowing club with people half my age. Admirable, perhaps, but also foolhardy.

In 2004, in my second year of rowing, I had gone to see Dr. Sandra Parkhill, a rheumatologist, for a persistent deep ache in my upper right leg. I thought it was due to arthritis or inflammation in my sacroiliac joint. I had ignored it for a year.

"It's not your sacroiliac joint," Dr. Parkhill said after she listened to my story. "It's your back. You almost certainly have a slipped disc. You have to stop rowing." This problem had nothing to do with my Parkinson's and everything to do with the limitations of self-diagnosis and my delay in seeking treatment. An MRI showed that Dr. Parkhill was quite right. I had a large protruding disc in my lower spine, sitting smack dab on some major nerve roots in the area. For the next year and a half I tried every remedy for the pain, and still it got worse, shooting down my right leg when I walked or with any pressure on my right foot. I had to take increasingly hefty doses of narcotics for even modest relief.

On one nasty night in the winter of 2005, when the pain medication was particularly ineffective, my wife took me to the ER. The neurosurgeon on call that night was very accommodating.

"Any time you want it fixed, just let me know."

Surgery for slipped discs—the removal of the arc of bone over the offending disc and the excision of the protruding portion of the disc—is one of the most common operations performed in North America. However, the actual value of the surgery for relief of *back* pain is questionable; it is better suited for relief of extremity pain. For 90 per cent of patients with back pain, the pain will go away with or without treatment. Those who opt for surgery may have more immediate relief but will later experience more chronic back pain on account of the surgery itself. I focused on the promise of immediate relief from my persisting and intolerable leg pain. I didn't resist the neurosurgeon's offer and had my first back surgery several months later. *No big deal*, I thought, *just a little operation.*

For a short while after the operation, I did feel much better. After a few months, though, the pain returned. I felt embarrassed, ungrateful almost, having to go back to have a second operation the next year. And then I had yet another operation. One of the bones in my back had fractured (likely during that second operation) and was sliding back and forth over the vertebra below, squeezing a spinal nerve root. This third surgery was a back fusion, which limited my flexibility, but seemed unavoidable.

The relief that followed the operation was, however, temporary. Over the next half year, the pain intensified and my legs weakened. I had to crawl up my front steps. I was regularly admitted to the hospital for pain relief. On one occasion, I was experiencing pain unlike any I had before. At home, thoughts of suicide danced in my head. I was admitted to hospital for pain relief. My leg felt as if it was on fire and being crushed at the same time. I had insufficient relief from the medications the night nurse administered and I had to ring for help. My nurse seemed annoyed.

"You had your pain medication less than an hour ago."

"Maybe, but I'm in agony!"

"You are on the same dose you were on when you were discharged. It should be enough."

"But my pain is worse now. The same dose isn't working."

The nurse was disinclined to give me more pain medication. "You aren't due for more for at least another hour."

I tried to stay calm but I doubt that I was. I probably was hysterical. I felt that I was losing this argument. "But I can't wait that long!"

The nurse gave me a cold stare. "Well, you'll just have to. Don't bother ringing for anyone else. I'm going on break and no one else will give you more. You've had enough." With that, she turned around and left.

After she was gone, I cried and cried out. No one came. I was terrified. Perhaps my recollection is skewed by the pain I was in, perhaps she couldn't do anything more, perhaps it would have been dangerous to give me more drugs. She may have been right. But what made me most distressed was being left alone. As health care professionals we sometimes forget that, even if we cannot fix a problem, we can stay with our patients, talk to them, provide a kind and compassionate presence. When my wife visited later that evening, she was horrified by my story. She went away and found my surgeon and dragged him back to my room. He, too, was upset with my care and ordered more pain medication. Yet my ongoing pain perplexed him. He asked for a colleague's advice. The two surgeons agreed on one thing: no further surgery. If three didn't help, they thought a fourth would make me worse. I received various opinions, none in favour of surgery. "Wait. Tough it out." "Give it a few more months." "Perhaps it will get better on its own." "Maybe you're just constipated." If these surgeons couldn't help me, who could?

By the late fall of 2006, I felt like a drowning man searching for a lifeline, so I pulled some strings. I put in a call to a colleague and friend in neurosurgery at another hospital. I remembered he had driven himself from his cottage to his own hospital after a spinal injury and had been successfully operated on there. "Dr. Verne is our best," he told me. "I'll speak to him today about you."

Several days later I went to see Dr. Verne in his office. He seemed an impressive, confident surgeon. Quickly looking over the latest MRI of my back, he said to me, "Your fusion didn't take. You need a re-do. I can help you," he said. He agreed to operate on me straight away. I was set up for urgent back surgery. I felt so relieved I almost cried. Two days later, I had a fourth back surgery.

After the seven-hour surgery I didn't wake up as expected. My body was rigid, my blood pressure dangerously elevated, and when I did wake up, I was delirious. I felt suffocated, as though I were underwater, paralyzed. I looked around but had no idea who—or where—I was. Wherever I was, there were people wandering around, looking like aliens with strange masks and shining headlamps. They seemed able to walk on walls and up and down perpendicular staircases, defying gravity, like an Escher drawing. I was obviously hallucinating but it seemed all too real to me.

My wife appeared on the scene, having also walked up the wall. "Philip," she said, "there were some complications and you are in the ICU."

As I woke up from my drug-induced stupor, so did my back. The pain was relentless. Thank goodness for the administrations of morphine. The drug's name derives from Morpheus, the god of sleep. But he's a crafty character. According to Ovid, he can take any form. He can induce narcosis and sleep. He can also cause hallucinations and agitation.

I was moved to a step-down unit. For several more days my mind continued to play tricks on me. My bed became my car and I kept crashing into snow banks. Everything tasted and smelled awful: meat like sawdust, water like plastic. Scents were intensified to an intolerable level. The floor seemed to be made of fire, ice, and broken glass. I made a dash for the elevator. Two burly guards escorted me back to my hospital room. They would be with me for days.

Eventually, my senses slowly began to return to normal. I calmed down, recognized that I was in a hospital, recuperating from another round of back surgery. The burly guards were actually nurses.

"Boy, I sure am loopy, aren't I?"

My wife did not disagree. "When you didn't wake up from surgery, they thought you'd had a stroke. A CAT scan ruled that out. You've also had a ton of morphine— enough to kill a horse!"

My delirium had mistakenly been thought by the residents to be what's known as ICU psychosis, a psychotic state associated with prolonged complicated surgery, and they treated it, as they almost always do, with haloperidol.

My wife happens to know more than a little about my medications and about pharmacology, and she knew that the haloperidol should be stopped. While the drug is effective for many patients, it was an unfortunate choice for anyone with Parkinson's; it lowered my already diminished dopamine levels, making a bad situation even worse. But she found it hard to intervene. She did not want to overexert her expertise. But she also knew the residents had based their actions on pattern recognition. Rather than investigating why I might be delirious, they assumed they knew why and treated me according to the protocol they had learned. My wife gently suggested that they might want to consider an alternative treatment to haloperidol and that they might administer its usual anti-dote. They agreed. But it seems they ordered too much of the antidote, which deepened my confused state.

I shudder to think what would have happened had my wife not been a physician and recognized the error of haloperidol having been administered to me. What would have happened to someone who did not have such an expert advocate? My delirium had in part been caused by the huge doses of morphine I had been receiving. But the surgery itself had been hastily arranged. As in football, it was a kind of Hail Mary pass, one done on a hope and a prayer, with little chance of success. Perhaps because of the hurried-up transfer to a different hospital just before the surgery, inadvertently I was not given my usual Parkinson's medications at the proper times. Lack of those drugs caused a precipitous drop in my brain's dopamine levels. The sudden drop in dopamine resulted in what is known as neuroleptic malignant syndrome, a life-threatening state of confusion, which manifests as extreme agitation and muscular rigidity. That was the ori-gin of my high blood pressure and my sense of paralysis.

In 2004, I had participated, in a small way, as a co-author of the Canadian Adverse Events Study, the first national study of surgical and drug-related errors in Canadian hospitals. The study revealed a hidden epidemic of medical error. We estimated that, in the year 2000, roughly 9,000 to 24,000 deaths from medical errors were preventable.[2] Two years later, my own situation would, ironically, fall within the very category we had studied. Are unwanted outcomes of care unavoidable and random, like earthquakes and meteors? Usually not, and not in my case. Perhaps the staff were so focused on getting my back surgery right that they paid less mind to other aspects of my care, and so had failed to make sure my other medications were ordered at the right times and in proper doses.

For years afterwards, I would easily be brought to tears just thinking of these events and my time in the ICU. I realize now that I was suffering from a kind of post-traumatic stress reaction. Although all of the staff tried to help me with my delirium, I never received a good explanation or an apology for what had transpired. Admittedly, at the time it didn't matter. As with many patients, I wanted to concentrate on getting better.

Certainly, when medical errors and unexpected outcomes of care do happen, patients and families should expect timely and proportionate responses from health care professionals. Besides learning from these events in order to prevent them, medical practitioners should respond to patients' expectations of an open disclosure. The more serious the event, the more prompt and thorough that response should be. And apologies should go along with such transparency.

Unfortunately, my back did not get better as predicted. I had to undergo two more back fusion surgeries in the next three years, the last one in 2009. I was much improved, but, as is to be expected after six back surgeries, my back would never be the same. Hurried-up care or more surgical care is not necessarily better care.

Meanwhile, my Parkinson's disease had progressed. I would have brief periods when I would freeze and be unable to leave an examining room to attend to other patients. I found myself unable to do proper breast or abdominal examinations, as they require coordinated rotational hand movements that at times I could not manage. At other times a tremor appeared to interfere with my dexterity and ability to do simple procedures such as joint injections. My balance was failing as well; I was unable to carry a cup in each hand at the same time. Although for a while my medications had helped, my handwriting went downhill. More than once I had to help pharmacists decipher my handwritten prescriptions. I tried to deflect any criticism by joking that bad handwriting was a required course in medical school.

But most worrying of all I was distracted by my illness. Some days it was hard to focus, hard to listen to my patients. I felt much sicker, more impaired even on good days, than many of my patients, many of whom were much older than I was. I thought this was my secret.

Then one day Mrs. Sadie Sampson came in to see me. Sadie was in her mid-eighties; she was on several medications and had a chart as thick as a brick. Macular degeneration had made her almost blind. Heart failure and emphysema weighed upon her chest like a stone.

"I don't breathe as well as I used to, Doctor, but I'm fine. Really, I am. I can get around," Sadie said. Her chest had the usual crackles, her blood pressure was low but acceptable, her ankles were swollen, also usual for her. We tinkered a little with her medications. Then, as Sadie, almost blind and barely able to catch her breath, was leaving my office, she turned to me and said, "Now, Doctor, tell me: what's wrong with your leg?"

I mumbled something about an old war wound, but I could tell she knew I was being coy. It suddenly dawned on me: If *she* could tell something was amiss, so could everyone else. Who did I think I was fooling?

With each of my surgeries, I had promised my patients I would soon be back. But each recovery took longer than the one before. After my sixth back surgery, I wouldn't be able to keep my promise: I would have to be off work for at least a year. My Parkinson's was only getting worse.

I would no longer be able to do the things doctors do: take a blood pressure, try to solve a difficult patient problem, or even just listen to a patient's story. I didn't think I had any cognitive impairments. But I was still on large doses of analgesics and could barely negotiate the path to my clinic from the parking lot because of my back pain and stiff gait. Most disturbingly, my illness *diverted* me from the tasks at hand. I did not want to stay in practice if I could not do so at what I considered an exemplary and comprehensive level. So in 2010, I made one of the hardest decisions of my life—I decided to retire from active medical practice. I considered my patients to be my friends. I owed them an explanation for my inability to remain their doctor. Telling them individually seemed too hard. Instead, I sent out a letter to all my patients acknowledging my Parkinson's and its progression. I hoped for a quiet exit.

Could I have told my patients earlier? Yes, I think so. They would have understood my illness. *Should* I have told them earlier? Only if I was putting them at risk by continuing to practice. Who would be the judge of that, however?

The potential for a conflict between my private life—Parkinson's and my ongoing back troubles, which required high doses of narcotics—and my professional roles—as a family doctor and an ethics consultant—was never far from the surface, I would have to say, but, as a conflict, it was not new. Medical trainees, for example, are often faced with a conflict between their educational needs and the well-being of patients. How much experience does a trainee need before he or she can safely perform a procedure on a patient? Do they need to get consent from a patient before drawing blood or inserting a chest tube for the first time? What about the first time residents do surgical incisions on their own?

Medical students are carefully supervised when doing such work, as they should be. A mentor is there to guide and to steady the inexperienced hand and to soothe the worried patient. Trainees are typically young and enthusiastic, so although the learning curve may be steep, they have a capacity to learn that is usually equal to the task at hand. They are also, generally, well. The situation is quite different for doctors such as myself, impaired by illness, whose capacity to learn will certainly be diminished—diminished not just by age but also by the absence of appropriate oversight. In most jurisdictions, physicians have not been required to disclose their own failings or those of their colleagues (unless the behaviour pertains to sexual impropriety with patients, which must be reported to the doctor's regulatory authorities in all circumstances).

With an increased concern for patient safety, however, the situation may be changing. "League tables" listing individual physicians' patient outcomes (deaths, readmission rates, complication rates, patient satisfaction scores) are released in the U.K. and in a number of American states. Regulatory authorities in Canada, Australia, and the United States increasingly require doctors to report when they have a medical condition that may affect their ability to practise. In some places it is left to physicians to impose a "fitness to practise" standard on themselves. In other places there is a requirement to report on impaired colleagues—much like commercial airline pilots are reported (or should be) if they have a condition that affects their ability to fly safely. The safety of so many others depends on this.

I could deny the impact of my conditions on my ability to function for only so long. In the conflict between the patient's well-being and a physician's wish to continue practising, the patient's interests must win out.

It was only as the five-hour operation proceeded—with me awake the whole time, my skull cut open—that I was finally convinced, once and for all, that I had Parkinson's.

During the procedure a neural probe—a tiny wire, barely thicker than a human hair, with four electrodes at the end—was passed through my brain to its base and connected to a neurostimulator in my chest. During the surgery, my surgeon, Dr. Misra, had me perform tasks with my left arm and leg, the most affected parts of me. A team was "interrogating" individual neurons, or nerve cells, to make sure they were in the right place, that being my *globus pallidus*, the "pale globe" of brain cells that, along with conjoined neurons at the brain's base, enables smooth voluntary movements, learning, and emotional expression. Over the speakers in the operating room I could hear my neurons busily chatting amongst themselves, a cacophony of static. Several hours into the operation, suddenly I felt different—released, looser. I knew right away that the neural probe was in the right place. My tremor disappeared. My left foot and leg could move more easily than they had for twenty years. My tears continued, but now they were tears of joy, not fear.

After the surgery I regained a good measure of my ability to walk. I had forgotten how effortless it can be! How long the benefit of the deep brain stimulation will last is impossible to predict. For now, the neurodegenerative process of Parkinson's continues but in a hidden way. I have never been so aware of my own mortality and of the preciousness of life.

Being a patient has been, for me, the roughest schooling of all. The uncertainties and the pain I experienced, the medications I took, the surgeries I had were all tougher than I could ever have imagined. I have received, and benefited from, the best of medical care. I have also received less than optimal care and delayed care—sometimes of my own making, sometimes on account of systemic errors. I have learned that more care isn't always better care. And I have learned that nothing can replace careful, caring practitioners. Even when health care practitioners cannot solve a patient's problems, they can try to understand their patients better. There is also an important role for consoling, or for simply spending time with, the patient.

And, not surprisingly, while I encourage people to avail themselves of the best medical care possible, I also encourage a healthy skepticism of the latest medical fads. And I encourage taking great caution when it comes to even minor surgery.

Good medicine is a combination of having empathic professionals and, sometimes, just plain luck. Uncertainty and complexity certainly exist in all aspects of health care, which makes both providing and receiving good medical care very challenging.

That does not mean that patients and families should not expect it.

IV

THE PATIENT'S VOICE

Mary Czvok and I have been friends for many years. She is a sixty-three-year-old professor of political theory, married to Peter Ferris, a lawyer who is also an old friend of mine. They have two grown kids. One day in 2013 we were comparing medical horror stories, as people our age are prone to do. Mary's problems had seemed simple at first, but, slowly, inexorably, they turned out to be much more complicated than anyone had anticipated.

Sometime over the summer of 2011, Mary began to feel unwell. At first she thought the malaise was caused by an unusually hot summer or perhaps was some late menopausal effect. She was near retirement age. She wasn't sure how a person in her sixties was supposed to feel. At any rate, Mary had better things to think about—her students, her family, and a book she was writing on Gramsci, the Italian revolutionary who died at a young age after being imprisoned by Mussolini in the 1930s. Besides, Mary said, some days she felt quite well. On others, though, it was a chore just to get out of bed. Over several months, her desire for sex and even for food diminished. Peter was worried she was depressed and encouraged her to see her doctor.

But Mary didn't feel depressed, and she continued to ignore her symptoms. Then, late in 2011, she woke up to find a few red spots on her torso. Over the next two weeks they spread to her limbs and became itchy. She thought she might be allergic to something. For several weeks she eliminated things she thought might be triggering the reaction—a new lotion she had used, her soap, her deodorant—but the rash got worse. Scratching and antihistamines provided no relief; the rash became uncomfortably itchy and kept her awake at night.

She called Dr. Paul Fowler, her family physician, the only doctor she had seen for years. He was informal and very welcoming but not rigorous. Many considered him their friend as much as their doctor. Dr. Fowler exuded a sense of confidence, but more than one patient had expressed concerns about his diagnostic acumen. Mary was among the dissatisfied. But she hadn't needed to see him very often and so hadn't got around to changing doctors.

Nothing urgent about a rash, his booking clerk decided, giving her an appointment in two weeks' time. By then, work and concentration had become difficult.

When she saw Dr. Fowler, she mentioned that she thought the glands in her neck were enlarged. He examined her but didn't make much of this concern.

"You have a few shotty nodes in your neck," he said, meaning, in medical terms, small, hard nodes that felt like buckshot. They were not tender or terribly enlarged, in his estimation.

As for the rash, noting its concentration on her limbs, he was again a bit dismissive. "Maybe you have bedbugs."

That, thought Mary, *is gross*. She and Peter were phobic about insects, all flurries of legs and waving antennae. Besides, Peter didn't have a rash. Why would the bedbugs only go after her?

Mary was back in Dr. Fowler's office later that month. "Just send me to someone! We don't have bedbugs. Nor do we have fleas."

As with all patients in Canada, unless Mary was prepared to go though an emergency room, she had to be referred to a specialist by her family physician. However, asking Dr. Fowler for a referral was like pulling teeth. Many family doctors now have financial incentives to look after all the needs of their patients, minimizing expensive after-hour visits to emergency rooms and reliance on specialist care. Patients, though, may have to wait an inordinately long time to see a specialist. Mary thought Dr. Fowler took his role as gatekeeper to the health care system too seriously. He was more of a gate-closer than a door-opener. *I really should find another doctor*, she thought at the time, but even in the large metropolitan arc of Greater Toronto, finding a good doctor with openings is not always easy. Anyway, Dr. Fowler was not a *uniformly* bad doctor; sometimes he listened well and could tell a funny joke.

With a little pressure and persistence from Mary and Peter, Dr. Fowler agreed to send her to a dermatologist in private practice, Dr. Elizabeth Curtis. Mary saw her early in 2012. Dr. Curtis examined Mary and found nothing unusual about the rash. She told Mary she had what is known as neurotic eczema, a skin inflammation of unknown cause. It is thought to be exacerbated by emotional issues. It is also considered a "diagnosis of exclusion," one that should be entertained only when more serious causes have been excluded.

"Are you having any troubles at home?" Dr. Curtis asked. Mary guessed the doctor was doing her best to consider her as a whole person, psyche as well as soma.

"Not at all." *Everybody has issues. Not everybody gets a rash*, Mary thought.

Dr. Curtis prescribed an anti-inflammatory cortisone cream. It didn't work. The other creams and emollients that Mary was prescribed on subsequent visits were not very helpful either. They alleviated the itch a little, but her skin was now a patchwork of scratches.

"You've got to stop scratching yourself! Wear mittens at night," Dr. Curtis advised. "Get more rest. Exercise. Practise meditation."

Dr. Curtis seemed unable to help Mary. But she neither recommended any testing nor suggested Mary get a second opinion. And Mary didn't push it. She was not used to being ill and trusted her doctors to be thorough.

Back in Dr. Fowler's office a few months later, Mary again mentioned her swollen neck glands and the still-unresolved rash. Dr. Fowler was facing away from her, busily entering notes in Mary's chart on a fancy computer. "Your neck glands are a little enlarged—likely that's from a virus." He leaned back in his chair and seemed to smile a little. Now she could make eye contact with him.

Is he trying to be reassuring or funny? Either way, Mary started to get annoyed.

"I don't remember having a virus or anything like that." She'd had it up to here with the rash and was close to tears. "Can't I see somebody else? Dr. Curtis is kind-hearted, but my rash has her stumped."

"He could see how upset I was," Mary told me. Dr. Fowler referred her to another dermatologist, this one in a teaching practice.

Before she could see him, however, Mary developed a second and *different* rash—a band of blisters around the right side of her waistline. It was painful, and uncomfortable with even a light touch. She diagnosed herself with shingles, something both her parents had had in their later years. Shingles is a recurrence of childhood-acquired chicken pox. It is more common in the elderly and those with reduced immunity. In retrospect it was an ominous warning.

Mary saw the second dermatologist, Dr. Russell James, in the late summer of 2012. The shingles had resolved by then, but her original rash was still bothersome. Dr. James took a superficial shave biopsy of her skin; it showed only some inflamed abnormal cells. He told Mary he concurred with the previous diagnosis of neurotic eczema and suggested she must have some hidden psychological issues. No follow-up was offered. Mary remembers Dr. James seeming more interested in showing his resident how to do the biopsy than he was in her.

After several more months of feeling no better, Mary pleaded with Dr. Fowler to send her to yet another specialist. Dr. Fowler had accepted the opinion of the "experts" about the rash and only reluctantly did he agree to the referral. "This is the last!" he warned her, without re-examining her himself.

So Mary saw Dr. Eva Wong—the fourth doctor— for her rash, in February 2013, a year and a half after the onset of her malaise. Dr. Wong looked too young to inspire much confidence. She had, however, a serious demeanour, and she listened carefully to Mary's story.

Her eyes widened when Mary disrobed in the examining room. "Your skin really is awful! You must be suffering. How long has it looked this bad?" Eva peered at Mary's rash, now with scattered blisters on an angry-looking coalescence of red patches. Mary was embarrassed by her appearance and by how long she had tolerated the rash. But she was also pleased that someone was finally taking her seriously. "I don't know what you've been told, but this is not eczema," Dr. Wong said. "I'm pretty certain I know what this is. To be sure, I'll have to take a deeper skin biopsy than you've had and get some blood work done as well."

Mary returned to Dr. Wong a week later. The biopsy had revealed her rash was dermatitis herpetiformis, an uncommon rash that occurs in people with gluten sensitivity. Mary's immune system, triggered by gluten in her intestines, was attacking her skin. Mary would have to follow a strict gluten-free diet and she would need to be on medication for some months. Dr. Wong warned her about the drug, which, as it happens, is also used to treat leprosy. Some people are unpredictably sensitive to the drug and get a very serious skin condition called Stevens-Johnson syndrome in reaction to it. The condition can be life-threatening. Dr. Wong warned Mary to call her right away if she felt worse in any way. "If I am unavailable, go to the ER," she added.

The good news is that I don't have leprosy, Mary thought. *Or herpes. The bad news is the treatment might kill me.* But Mary was so desperate to get better that she would have taken anything at that point.

After she began treatment, Mary's persistent rash rapidly resolved. Yet she did not feel as well as she hoped she would. She was still profoundly listless. She had been losing weight, and the swellings in her neck were clearly more pronounced. Mary was sure the lymph nodes in her groin were now swollen as well. She had paid less attention to these symptoms when her rash was at its zenith. And now she had developed a new symptom: severe and relentless back pain. She returned to her family doctor.

"You likely have a slipped disc," Dr. Fowler told her, adding, "X-rays are only recommended if the pain persists." He prescribed anti-inflammatory pills and strong pain medication. "Do you want to see our physiotherapist? She might help you." Dr. Fowler frowned when Mary declined to do so.

Mary tried to consider her situation objectively. Perhaps she was psychosomatic. She wondered if she was getting paranoid about her health. She was feeling so out of sorts, so lacking in energy, that she considered applying for long-term disability. This required her family doctor to complete a four-page form. Dr. Fowler told her quite frankly that she would likely not be eligible. He seemed sympathetic to her situation but said his hands were tied— she hadn't been diagnosed with a "serious disorder." He had missed the gluten-allergy thing, he admitted, but on its own it would not be enough to disable her from work.

Mary returned soon after to see Dr. Wong, who examined her swollen lymph nodes. She apologized for not having done so sooner, saying, "You've got bigger issues than the dermatitis." Dr. Wong called a senior hematologist, Dr. John Darcy, knowing that if the call came directly from her, Mary would get an urgent appointment. She had been a resident with Dr. Darcy and knew he thought highly of her. Indeed, Dr. Darcy agreed to see Mary the next day. Mary was anxious about this referral and yet also relieved. Her concerns and worries had been acted upon promptly.

Dr. Darcy exuded a calm and professional manner. His office was on an upper floor of a large teaching hospital and had a commanding view of downtown Toronto. After thoroughly examining Mary and chatting a little, he got down to business. "As Dr. Wong noted, you have unusually enlarged lymph nodes everywhere. Your spleen is also a lot bigger than it should be. I don't know what, but something besides gluten is stimulating your immune system and causing your lymph nodes to be swollen. We need to get to work right away and figure out what's going on. At this point I'm unsure what's causing your back pain. It is likely related to whatever is making you feel so ill." He said he would order some tests but it would take two weeks to get back definitive results.

Mary didn't want to wait that long; she wanted to be prepared for what was coming. Gramsci's fortitude emboldened her. One of his teachings was well known but ill understood: "Pessimism of the intellect, optimism of the will." She would need to know what difficulties she faced and somehow find the will, the spirit, to overcome them.

"Doctor, can you please tell me what possibilities you are considering?" Mary glanced at her husband, who had taken time off work to be with her.

"Are you sure you want to know? Some are quite serious and they are all, at this point, just possibilities."

Managing to nod yes, Mary suddenly felt the room closing in around her. She held her breath and grasped for Peter's hand.

"Well, your symptoms and findings are most suggestive of some type of lymphoma, a cancer of the immune system."

Recently, Mary had sensed that she was much sicker than anyone had thought. And she was right. *Oh, my God. Now Dr. Fowler will have a good reason to complete my damn disability form* was all she could think.

The hematologist ordered blood tests, X-rays, a CT scan, an ultrasound, an MRI, and biopsies of her swollen lymph glands. He also arranged for her to see an oncologist. By June 2013, the cause of Mary's enlarged lymph nodes was finally uncovered: an advanced and slow-growing form of non-Hodgkin's lymphoma. A large lymphoma-related mass was pressing on her spinal cord. Her fatigue, weight loss, malaise, back pain, and likely the shingles were all manifestations of the lymphoma. Her long-standing rash seemed to have been a red herring. The attention of most of the doctors had been focused on it while her real problem lay elsewhere.

The oncologist was reassuring. Even advanced lymphomas like Mary's are treatable, he said, and, if a permanent cure is not possible, then at least a remission for some years almost always is. This was a lot of difficult information for Mary and Peter to absorb. Neither of them knew much about illness or cancer. They would have a lot to learn. The oncologist was honest. The treatment he was recommending would not be pleasant. Mary would have to steel herself. The dull and pressing weight of her new reality, that she was seriously ill, settled over her. Gramsci's maxim took on a renewed and deeper meaning.

Dr. Fowler completed Mary's disability form. He admitted his errors in her care and apologized for being too cavalier and not taking her seriously. She accepted his apologies with graciousness.

Mary's treatment started in late summer, and her chances for long-term cure improved. From start to finish, however, it had taken Mary *more than two years* and seeing *five* doctors to receive a proper diagnosis and effective care.

Today Mary is doing reasonably well. Her blood counts have gone up and down and her lymph nodes have shrunk. Fatigue remains a major issue but at times she feels like her old self.

But for me, her story is a sad and distressing one. Sad because it took my friend so long to be properly diagnosed. And distressing because the attitudes of some clinicians remain "old school" and obstructive to good medicine. The law cannot mandate good, comprehensive medical care. Medical ethics—how to know and do the right thing—have been taught to physicians and medical trainees for years. Yet how much better was Mary listened to than Jerry had been, thirty years earlier?

Part of the problem with medicine in Canada is, at times, its slowness to change, its disorganization, and its lack of responsiveness to the concerns of patients. Mary's care would have been better had her health care providers been better organized, had they utilized modern technology more expeditiously and talked more openly and seriously with each other as well as with Mary. In this case, the listening skills of doctors left much to be desired. Clearly communicating to patients the truth about their diagnoses and prognoses, especially with uncommon conditions, is a difficult and error-prone skill. But most diagnoses—at least 80 per cent of them, it has been said—can be made simply by talking with a patient, not by using fancy tests or procedures. This is an issue of how health care providers conduct ourselves with others. It raises the importance both of taking a patient's symptoms seriously and of being prepared to explore other diagnoses when the patient does not improve as we expect.

There is a valuable role for patients' families here. Perhaps Peter might have accompanied Mary to more of her appointments. He might have trusted his intuitions that his wife was more ill than anyone had suspected and communicated his concern more forcefully to her various doctors, urging them to take Mary's issues more seriously. Health care professionals cannot always be relied upon not to make mistakes. Thus, the necessary corrective role for patients and their families.

What Mary's first practitioners failed was the "empathy exam." They did not imagine themselves in her situation, ask about what her life was like, how her symptoms were affecting her and those around her. Empathic skills are fragile skills that can be eroded by cynicism and the demands of a busy practice. Currently, there are too few encouragements or opportunities for improving the empathic skills of health professionals once their training is completed.

In Mary's case, most of her physicians missed the mark. They did not consider the more ominous conditions that can lurk behind persistent, seemingly benign symptoms. They failed to take into sufficient consideration symptoms that didn't fit with their diagnosis, such as her swollen nodes. And, perhaps most important, they did not *talk with* Mary and thereby come to realize that this wasn't the illness they thought it was. Mary's views about her condition were never elicited—and had they been, I doubt they would have been heard as no one was listening.

Unfortunately, in the struggle against disease, patients and doctors can seem to be on opposing teams, meeting on an uneven playing field that tips in favour of the health care professionals. Physicians are too prone to bend to pressures, mostly from government or other third party payers, to guard against the overuse of medical resources. At the same time, patients' access to needed care can be too readily limited. This does not mean that results like Mary's—late diagnoses, wrong treatments—favour, or were wanted by, her doctors. They truly did want to provide the best of care. But absent Mary having a stronger voice, theirs were the only ones being heard. Only Dr. Wong showed Mary the empathy she deserved.

It did not take the good doctor an inordinate amount of time or resources to figure out that Mary was seriously ill. "Know thy patient well." It is the mantra every physician should adopt.

A DEATH FORETOLD,
A DEATH UNFOLDS

A late-winter storm in 1992 had set my father to work clearing the snow from his front walk and driveway. He was never one to let things rest. When he wanted something done, it was done right away. And if *you* did it, but it didn't meet to his expectations, he would do it again himself. The lawn had to be mowed just so, the snow removed immediately upon falling. We teased him about his perfectionism, but that didn't stop him. He just kept going—until the day of the storm.

My mother told us later that she had been worried when she looked out the front window at the heavily falling snow. "He should have let the neighbours' kids do it," she said. "But you know your father. He was too proud to ask them." My father was in his mid-seventies and not in the best of shape, having acquired a substantial waistline when he quit smoking.

After he finished shovelling that morning, my father went inside for his usual bacon and eggs breakfast. Moments after sitting down to eat, he made a loud snoring noise, as if he had suddenly fallen asleep. From the kitchen my mother, a former nurse, saw him collapsed at the table. She thought he had had a cardiac arrest. She rushed over to find that he was breathing, but was passed out, and as limp as a rag doll. She recognized a stroke when she saw it. She immediately dialed 911, and within minutes an ambulance was there. The emergency rescue team bundled up my father and carted him off to the hospital in Kingston, Ontario.

My mother was right—he had had a stroke, and one of the worst kind, a cerebral hemorrhage, a large bleed within his brain. He was completely unresponsive.

My father's collapse was not entirely a surprise. In fact, it had been predicted almost forty-five years before.

My father, Neil, was born a century ago, in 1915, and my mother, Evelyn, five years later. They met in their hometown of Kingston before WWII. When the war was over, they married, stayed put, and had five kids.

My dad was in apparent good health until one fine day in the summer of 1948. He was out strolling with my mother when his right leg started twitching. Next, his right arm began to jerk, then, uncontrollably, his left side, and finally his whole body convulsed.

He fell to the ground, losing consciousness for several minutes. When he came to, he was groggy, his muscles had cramped up, and his mouth was dry. A sharp dresser, he was at first most upset that he had ripped the knees of his nice new trousers. My mother, who had just graduated as a nurse, recognized that my father had experienced an epileptic seizure. She took him off to see Dr. Evan Slaight.

Everyone in Kingston knew Dr. Slaight. He'd been overseas during the war and was now a general practitioner. General he was. He could deliver a baby in the middle of the night, perform an appendectomy in a country kitchen, hack off a gangrenous leg. (Or so it was said.) He never seemed to be in a hurry and always had time for drop-in patients. He saw my father that same day.

Dr. Slaight was familiar with neurology, too, having spent part of his training under a famous British neurologist, the eponymously named Dr. Brain. He said my father had experienced a Jacksonian march seizure—named after the neurologist who, in the 1860s, first described the typical progression though the patient's motor cortex of this type of brain excitation. Seizures of this type are initiated by neurons suddenly activated by a local irritation in the brain, and then the activation spreads, like a fire, to nearby neurons. The seizure typically starts in one limb, usually a leg or hand, on one side of the body and then "marches" upwards, until the patient's whole body is convulsing and the patient loses consciousness.

Dr. Slaight knew his limitations. As he told my parents, "The question is not what you have, but why you have it. That is for minds more talented than mine to say." My mother and father, however, doubted there was anyone more talented than Dr. Slaight. But they accepted his referral for my father to see a specialist.

Within a month, Dr. J. Clifford Richardson, a renowned neurologist, examined my father in his office in a beautiful art deco medical building in downtown Toronto.[1] After a careful clinical examination, the doctor placed his stethoscope against my father's temple; he could hear a deep rumble inside my father's skull, like the passage of a distant train. He explained that the sound was most probably due to what is called an arterial-venous malformation, or AVM, an abnormal tangle of blood vessels in the brain. It was this proliferative growth that had caused my father's seizures. One further test was required to confirm the diagnosis.

The pneumoencephalogram was developed in the early years of the twentieth century and continued to be used until the advent of the CAT scan in the 1970s. To carry out this procedure, my father's spinal canal was punctured with a needle and some spinal fluid removed and replaced with air. He was then strapped face down onto a gurney and spun around, distributing the air throughout his central nervous system. The lighter air heightens the contrast between the patient's blood and the denser brain tissue. X-rays of my father's brain and its abnormal circulatory structure were taken when he was in upside-down and sideways positions. As an unavoidable consequence, my father was left, like a seasick sailor, unsteady, nauseated, and retching. He had terrible headaches for months afterwards and would later say the test was almost as bad as, if not worse than, having an epileptic spell.

Dr. Richardson met with my parents afterwards to discuss the implications of his finding. Surgery was not feasible, he said, as my father's AVM was buried too deeply. Instead, he prescribed two drugs, phenytoin and phenobarbital. Although then relatively new, they should be, he promised, a reliable duo. The drugs were intended to prevent my father's seizures (and, generally, as it turns out, did so). Dr. Richardson then stood up, shook my parents' hands, and said good luck and goodbye.

As my parents were leaving the office, almost as an afterthought Dr. Richardson advised my father that his brain was "a little sensitive." He warned my father not to get overly tired or exert himself too much. AVMs could rupture at any moment—especially if the patient was under undue pressure.

"You can follow up with Dr. Slaight. I'll see you in a year."

And that was that. There was nothing else anyone could do about the AVM. My father would return to see Dr. Richardson every year or two until not long before the doctor's death in 1986.

My father couldn't know when the AVM would rupture—no one could—but one day it likely would and that would be the end of things. Living under this medical sword of Damocles induced in my parents a sort of fatalism. Not surprisingly, one of their favourite songs became Doris Day's "Que Sera, Sera," a fatalistic song if there ever was one. We all knew of my father's condition; he would very occasionally have a seizure if he forgot to take his pills or was extremely tired. But his condition was never the topic of conversation at dinner. We understood we were not to speak of it. To my father, the AVM was a taboo topic; to discuss it would be tempting fate.

On the day of the big snowfall, more than forty years after my father's first seizure, the predicted event finally happened. My mother stayed with him all day while staff bustled about the ER. She left in the late evening to call us. At home, another snowfall had erased my father's handiwork.

The morning after my father's collapse, I arrived at the hospital. My mother and one of my sisters were already there. We were surprised to find that, although still comatose, my father had been admitted to a regular ward and would not be transferred to the ICU. He had been deemed "inappropriate" for transfer. All he had in the way of medical support was an intravenous line that was slowly dripping saline solution into his system.

Not even a heart monitor. Someone on the floor—likely the attending doctor—had decided that more aggressive care would be of no medical benefit. I was amazed that this decision had been made without our input. Whose father was he, anyway?

Having seen his brain scan, the doctors were pessimistic. We were shown these images. They looked like film negatives. Where grey (his brain) was supposed to be, there was now a huge blob of white (the bleeding), expanding, crushing all that was before it.

My reaction to these images was one of cold shock, like having my face plunged into ice water. *This is bad, really bad*, I thought, but kept it to myself. I didn't want to be seen as a collaborator of the ward doctors. I needed to be my father's advocate and family's ally. I did admit to my mother and sister that things didn't look very good.

My mother at first hoped my father's coma might lift a little if he was admitted to the ICU. These patients are intubated (a breathing tube is inserted down the throat to keep the airway open), the pressure inside the skull is monitored, and every available bodily orifice is used to maintain their cardiovascular, respiratory, and renal circulations as long as possible—until they die or improve. By the next day my mother, my siblings, and I were all at my father's bedside. For so long we'd taken his survival for granted, choosing to overlook his AVM and the likely impact of its rupture.

"I didn't ever really think how terrible it would be," said my mother.

None of us did, not even me. I was acquainted with some fine neurosurgeons, but it had never occurred to me to ask them whether my father's AVM might have been amenable to modern treatment. In fact I don't recall ever even discussing the issue of surgery with my father. I worried now that I had failed him.

When I confided this later to my mother, she reminded me that Dr. Richardson had followed my father regularly for three decades. He would have sent him for a surgical opinion had that been appropriate. Anyway, she said Dad would never have agreed to an operation on his brain.

Now that his AVM had ruptured, we discussed whether we wanted my father's treatment to be escalated to more aggressive levels. What we saw was that for the moment my father was breathing on his own. He looked almost peaceful. Somehow I hoped that, if he was provided with intensive care, he could ride out this storm. But the doctors described the results of the bleeding in my father's brain as catastrophic. I was pretty sure they were right—I had seen the brain scan images for myself— yet I still encouraged my mother to get other opinions. I wanted to make sure we had done all we could before we let Dad go.

Two neurosurgeons independently confirmed the opinion of the ward doctors. The bleeding could not be stanched. It had already destroyed my father's higher brain.

His lower brain would be next as, over the next few days, the pressure built up inside his skull. Then, without support or intervention, his breathing and circulation would fail. It was clear to me now that my father would not improve.

On the second day of my father's coma, Dr. Fox, the senior internist responsible for his care, approached my mother. "I have some questions I need to ask you," he said. He was standing at the foot of my father's bed. He said that the doctors had not been able to do much for my father. "We all know how ill Neil is. I need to ask you this. How much longer do you want to continue life support? Do you want resuscitation CPR if his heart stops?"

Left unsaid were what ends these measures might achieve for my father. We should have asked, but didn't. Perhaps it was the doctor's detached tone that inhibited our response. But I knew what the answer would be: there was nothing that could be, or should be, done for my father.

My mother glanced at me, looking for direction, and then asked for time to discuss it.

Dr. Fox was already at the door. "Well, it's your call. Let me know what you decide."

A visit that seemed to come from out of nowhere ended as quickly as it had begun. Surprisingly, no one came to help us make this decision—no chaplain, no social worker, no ethicist. Perhaps my father's doctors assumed that because I was a doctor, we didn't need any help. Or maybe the hospital didn't offer any such service.

I was by now keenly aware that my father would die no matter what was done. It had been several days since his stroke, and he showed no signs of improvement. None of my siblings entertained any optimism about his prognosis. We all agreed, the faster death came, the better.

The internist's questions were not unexpected, if a bit too abrupt and expressed in too rote a way. The openness with which my father's condition was discussed constituted a huge—and in my mind positive—change for medicine. It was in stark contrast to my training in the early 1980s, when resuscitation decisions were discussed *sotto voce* and only among the staff, very rarely with families. Back then, not providing CPR seemed somewhat illicit. "No CPR" orders were pencilled in on the duty roster for the day and erased when the patient died—to avoid any hint that the patient's departure was hastened in any way.

Most of us will die not primarily on account of our *hearts* suddenly stopping, however, but on account of *other* conditions that overwhelm us—such as metastatic cancer or, as in my father's case, a huge stroke. *Everything* is failing, not the heart alone. In such circumstances, trying to restart an arrested heart is almost always futile. I did worry that if my father's team were instructed not to do "everything," they would do "nothing." I had seen it happen before: patients with a "No CPR" order on their chart treated as if they had a "no care at all" order. I knew it would be up to us, his family, to clarify just what care we expected for my father. I wanted to make sure that my father received proper nursing care. We did not want a "No CPR" order to mean the nurses and doctors should all of a sudden disappear. Attention would still be provided—attentive general hygiene and assiduous skin and mouth care. This was simply good medicine.

As a former no-nonsense head nurse, my mother was from the old school, when hospitals smelled of disinfectant, not of coffee, and nurses wore starched white uniforms and caps. She could make tough decisions. But the ones she was now being asked to make seemed too slippery, too modern. How could she deny medical support to her husband of a half-century when he lay there looking like he might wake up at any moment? How much treatment was just the right amount?

There was no way around the unpalatable truth: things couldn't be much worse for my father. He would never be the man, the father, the husband he had been—no oil painting, no silly banjo playing, no cooking Sunday morning breakfasts, no shovelling the walk clear of snow. There was so much about my father that would be missed. I was saddened at the thought of the conversations I would now never have with him. As with many of his generation, he had been a quiet man. I knew too little of him.

"Think about what Neil would have wanted," advised one experienced nurse.

This was, finally, the heart of the matter and the key for my mother—she knew what was important to my father. He would not have wanted to be kept alive, even were this possible, in some severely impaired state. My father had known he was living on borrowed time—each year, each month, each day the AVM didn't rupture was a gift.

Knowing when and how to let go is a lesson that is hard for us all—patients, families, and health care professionals—to learn. Once my father's values were acknowledged, though, answers to the internist's questions seemed conceivable. It *would* matter what decision my mother came to: my father could spend his last few days on earth tethered to lines and devices, or we could recognize the inevitability of his death and aim to ensure his comfort while he was still alive. Technology would not determine my father's outcome; *he* would—through us.

In the cold light of an unforgiving injury, we decided that my father's treatment would not be escalated. He was, nevertheless, well looked after. He lingered for several more days in his comatose state. We took turns at his bedside, talking and laughing about that for which he was loved, for which he would be missed. My father died quietly, his laboured breathing slowly weakening, his wife and his children present. He had not suffered.

Later that week, as we waited out the last of winter's exacting storms, we gathered at the family home, sharing my mother's famous peach pie. We marvelled at my father's endurance and his resistance to forecasting. We all agreed, as well, that the choices we had faced in my father's care might have been less troubling, less difficult, had he openly discussed them in advance.

"It was a different time when we were younger," our mother explained. "We didn't talk about such things. Anyway, we were too busy raising you kids to worry about something we couldn't change." *Que sera, sera.*

On Christmas Eve 1994, less than two years after my father's death, my mother confessed that she had not been herself. She had felt off balance and nauseated for several weeks. Her aging family physician, Dr. Slaight, said she had a problem with the balance centre of the inner ear. "Nothing to get anxious about." He gave her some pills, but they hadn't made any difference.

My mother's dizziness returned with a vengeance on Christmas morning, when some of my siblings and I were at her home in Kingston, where she lived alone. My mother said that she was "not ill, only lonely," missing my father. We were concerned enough to press-gang her into visiting the ER. Though she kept protesting that she was wasting everybody's time, the ER staff took her complaint seriously, examined her, and, to our relief, had a brain CAT scan taken. It was normal.

"You see," she said to us, "Dr. Slaight was right after all."

When she felt a bit better the next day, she agreed to come back with us to Toronto. There, my mother divided her time between my house and my sister's. Her sense of imbalance returned. It was so marked at times that she couldn't get out of bed. We insisted that she be assessed once more, this time by a trusted colleague in my clinic. My colleague found nothing of concern, but ordered some blood tests. All the results were unexceptional.

Then, a week after her arrival in Toronto, my mother announced to my sister Jan that one of our cousins was prepared to drive her back to Kingston.

"I haven't been sleeping well here." She had already packed her things. "I'll be perfectly fine. I just need to be in my own bed."

Jan called me. My wife was on the phone with her. "Mom's insisting on going home today. June's agreed to drive her." I picked up the extension.

"Will she be okay?" my wife asked.

"I dunno—she's not as dizzy, but she's been up at night. And for the past few days she's been talking to people I can't see—like she's hallucinating."

"I don't think she should be going anywhere."

Without delay, we took my mother to the ER of the hospital where I worked. I trusted the staff there and could visit her when I wasn't in clinic. I could also keep a close eye on her care. I felt reassured. *We'll get some answers, get fixed whatever needs to be fixed.* My mother did not appear confused in the ER. We were all feeling a little sheepish, wondering if we had overreacted. I was standing by the nursing station with Dr. Wright, the supervising ER Casualty Officer, whom I knew.

"She may not look so bad now," I told him, "but at night especially she's really loopy. And that's not like my mother."

Dr. Wright managed a faint smile. "Oh, she's not going anywhere. There's something going on, I just don't know what it is. Now we have to find her a bed!"

My mother had always seemed indestructible. Strong, an excellent athlete, a capable nurse, she had been the driving force in the household. She had hardly been sick a day in her life and both of her parents lived well into their nineties. She was only seventy-four. To see her in such a debilitated state was inconceivable to us.

In the next few days my mother's confusion became more pronounced. She thought she was at home and wondered why so many strangers were there. She ate little, was less active, spending more time in bed, and complained about headaches and dizziness. She seemed to be shrinking into the hospital bed, folding into herself.

Then she would brighten like a swimmer surfacing from a deep sea, and for a few moments our hearts would rally. Her condition puzzled all. The doctors ordered a brain MRI. It, too, was normal. As was a chest X-ray, an abdominal-pelvic ultrasound, a spinal tap, all her blood work.

I still staunchly assumed there must be some treatable, reversible reason for her fluctuating level of awareness. Surely she would rally and get better.

Instead, my mother got much sicker over the next two weeks. One morning when we went to see her, she could not be roused. She had lapsed into a coma.

"She's just asleep," said the nurse, who admitted she had not herself tried to wake her.

It took three spinal taps to find the cause of my mother's decline. The resident, almost triumphantly, exclaimed, "The last spinal tap was positive for malignant cells!" It meant my mother had cancer somewhere in her central nervous system. If so, *where*? Her scans were all normal.

The brain MRI was repeated, this time using what is called an enhancing agent, a chemical that will light up the quickly dividing cells characteristic of cancerous tissue. The enhancing agent revealed a deadly rim of abnormal cells—too thin to be seen on an ordinary brain scan or MRI—tightly wrapped around my mother's brain stem, invading its covering and gradually choking off the life centre of her brain. My mother had very rare but aggressive cancer, a lymphoma of the infection-fighting white blood cells in the covering of her brain. There was, we were told, no known treatment.

Such a confined area of the brain was involved. Was my mother being denied treatment on account of her age? By now she was unrousable almost all the time. "Couldn't *something* be done?" one of my brothers asked.

We discussed treatment options with her specialist— an experienced and fine hematologist, Dr. John Senn, who had started the ethics centre at our hospital in 1988 and who seemed to be always available, ready to answer any questions we might have. He was also not afraid to provide direction and a professional recommendation. He told us that the lymphoma's spread around the brain stem was so rapid and extensive that it made it unlikely that any treatment would be effective.

"If my spouse had this condition," Dr. Senn offered, "I wouldn't want her to have any treatment. What good would it do? You would not gain much, if anything."

As had been the case with my father, there were many decisions to be made. Should my mother receive intravenous fluids to prevent dehydration? What about cardiac resuscitation if her heart stopped? Should she be intubated, and should she be transferred to the ICU if she stopped breathing on her own?

Like my father, my mother didn't have a formal living will. But she didn't really need one. The point of living wills or advance directives should be to encourage conversations among family members and with health care practitioners about medical care so that patients may exert some control over their deaths. If patients cannot confirm their wishes in writing, they may do so orally. My father's death, altogether too recently, had prompted us to discuss with my mother her wishes in the event of an illness if she could not speak for herself. We knew very well what she wanted. She did not want to be kept alive should she have irreversible mental incapacity, should her illness be terminal.

My mother was, as my father had been, "overmastered" by illness. Doing things that are ordinarily provided to the critically ill—providing IV fluids, artificial breathing support, or CPR—would not be appropriate for her. Her heart and her breathing stopping on account of her brain's functional failure seemed a natural way to go, all things considered.

Without regaining consciousness, my mother died just over one week later, with all of us, her family, beside her. And, as with my father, she received the best of care that good medicine could provide. In the face of a terrible, irremediable, and unexpected illness, she was able to exert a measure of control and was allowed to die in as unobstructed a way as could be hoped for.

THE QUALITY OF OUR MERCY

Not long after arriving in Canada from Iran in 2010, fifty-eight-year-old Hassan Rasouli began to complain to his wife of hearing loss. Several months later, doctors found a small benign tumour in his brain, behind his right ear. His wife, Parichehr Salasel, was worried, but not Hassan. He never worried about such things. He let Parichehr do his worrying for him. Hassan just wanted the problem fixed.[1]

Parichehr, Hassan, and their two children had left an increasingly religious Iran to secure the futures of their son and daughter. Hassan and Parichehr, each in their fifties when they left Iran, were well educated; he was an engineer and she had been a primary care doctor.

When Hassan's tumour was discovered, he was referred to a neurosurgeon in Toronto, where he and

Parichehr lived. Hassan and his wife considered the surgeon to be suitably confident. "In two days, three days at most, he'll be home," the surgeon told them. "The operation Hassan needs is not a big problem, believe me."

They did believe him, and they agreed to let the surgeon operate on Hassan's brain. A surgical consent form was obtained and the necessary paperwork completed. It seemed like a rather routine procedure, hardly risky at all. Indeed, the operation went well, and the tumour was removed.

But almost exactly three years later, in October 2013, Hassan and his family were at the centre of a case before the Supreme Court of Canada, fighting to keep Hassan on life support against the opinion of his doctors in that same hospital. Although the case would be decided upon a statutory interpretation of Ontario's Health Care Consent Act, within public discourse it would raise questions about who should have the ultimate say in end-of-life decisions. As Chief Justice Beverley McLachlin wrote in the majority judgment in favour of Hassan's family, "This case presents us with a tragic yet increasingly common conflict. A patient is unconscious. He is on life support—support that may keep him alive for a very long time, given the resources of modern medicine. His physicians, who see no prospect of recovery and only a long progression of complications as his body deteriorates, wish to withdraw life support. His wife, believing that he would wish to be kept alive, opposes withdrawal of life support. How should the impasse be resolved?"[2]

It wasn't supposed to turn out like this.

When it comes to serious illness, each family reacts differently when trying to find the right balance between acceptance and hope. Culture and religion, as well as personal convictions, affect how we make tough decisions for and about our loved ones. I hoped, as an outside ethics consultant, to better understand, if only for myself, the issues at the centre of Hassan's story from the point of view of his family; a point of view that had not, I felt, been well presented by the media.

I met with Parichehr and her two children at the hospital in October 2014, four years after Hassan's surgery and ten months after the Supreme Court released its ruling. Hassan was a patient at Sunnybrook Health Sciences Centre, where I had once been the chair of the Research Ethics Board. (I was never involved in Hassan's care and have had no access to his chart.)

According to his family, Hassan's problems began right after the operation. Parichehr told me, "They let me see him briefly when he came out of the OR. He was awake, sleepy of course, but he responded to me. He gave me a thumbs-up. I thought he was okay." That was the last time she was able to clearly communicate with him.

Shortly after, when the medical team tried to remove Hassan's breathing tube, for some reason they were unable to do so. They attempted to replace the tube in the recovery room. It did not go well. Parichehr says she was told that in the process her husband's oxygen levels may have fallen. Hassan had a heart attack and suffered a deep stroke in his right brain, which paralyzed his left side. "I saw what had happened to Hassan and I couldn't believe it," Parichehr said. "Could this really happen in a country like Canada?" She and Hassan knew that Canadian health care was good, but she missed aspects of the Iranian system, a system she knew intimately. She finds fault in a lack of continuity of care providers in this country.

"Surgeons in Iran," she told me, "follow their own patients from the time of surgery and for all the time afterwards while the patient is in the hospital. Here, it seemed like the doctors changed every few days. Sometimes I didn't know who they were." For Parichehr, this created communication problems.

There was unlikely to have been as much discontinuity as Parichehr perceived, but her confusion is understandable. At Sunnybrook, as at most hospitals in Canada, surgeons follow their own patients after surgery. In teaching hospitals, the surgical fellows and residents, who may see the patient most frequently and develop a rapport with the family, do change every month or two. The lead physician on the ward or in the ICU—the "attending"—might change weekly or monthly. Many other physicians, not to speak of allied health professionals, would also have been involved in Hassan's care. For every patient in the ICU, there are large multidisciplinary meetings, or rounds, to minimize the risks associated with discontinuity. I cannot say whether this was all explained to Hassan's family, but it would be unusual if it was not. Nonetheless, it was Parichehr's perception of discontinuity that was important, as it affected how strongly she and her family reacted to proposed limitations to Hassan's care.

After Hassan's deterioration in the recovery room, he was transferred to the ICU. "It was so hard for them to put the breathing tube down his throat. Maybe they damaged the covering of his airway. Maybe bacteria would spread from there to his brain." Parichehr pleaded with the staff to continue her husband's antibiotics, but she was resisted, she says. She is not sure why.

Parichehr told me she felt helpless. In Iran she would have been more directly involved in Hassan's care. Here, perhaps because of language and cultural differences, or maybe because she was a woman, she felt she was not taken seriously. She had no medical sway. Perhaps, she speculated, Hassan's doctors thought she was overreacting. Parichehr admitted that she was upset some days. She tried to be polite with and respectful of staff, despite the differences she had with them over Hassan's care. But Parichehr was determined to get her way—to keep her husband alive at all costs. She was not one to be easily placated or readily ignored.

After a week in the ICU, and still barely responsive, Hassan developed a fever. He was diagnosed with pneumonia. Then, most worryingly, he developed bacterial meningitis. He became deeply comatose and could not be roused at all. His wife and children say they had seen this train coming down the track—they are sure that the brain infection was a consequence of the surgery and just as sure that if the antibiotics had been continued, it could have been avoided. This is a disputed issue. Meningitis is a recognized risk any time the brain is opened to the air, and that would have been—or should have been—explained before Hassan consented to the surgery. In any case, continuing to administer antibiotics would have been of unlikely benefit and would have had its own risks, such as allergic or sensitivity reactions or the overgrowth of antibiotic-resistant infections.

In early 2011, after he had been on life support for four months, Hassan was diagnosed as being in what is called a persistent vegetative state. Part of his brain stem was at least partially functioning, and thus some of his bodily reflexes were preserved. Patients in this condition may open their eyes from time to time but cannot really "see." Nothing would register in their brains, and so, it is thought, no sensory input would occur, no willed action would be possible.

For doctors, the persistent vegetative state is an end-stage situation. Very few patients recover from it. There are no definitive tests for it, and so it is a clinical diagnosis that can be made only after many months of observation. (Those who do recover are often thought to have been wrongly or prematurely diagnosed in the first place.) Although patients in this state are almost always severely neurologically impaired, through assiduous care they can be kept alive for years. After being in the *persistent* state for anywhere from three months to a year, a patient is considered to be in a *permanent* vegetative state. For doctors, "permanent" means that a patient has crossed a line; there is *never* any going back. By the time I met with his family, Hassan had crossed that line.

Hassan's family has always maintained that he can still "treasure his life" even in this state. "Hassan's motto was, simply, be happy," his daughter, Mojgan, said. They believe he is happy in some way. His family favour life no matter how meagre its apparent quality. "It would be a different thing if he were in pain," Mojgan said. "But he's not."

Hassan's family is convinced he is still "in there," somewhere. They see movements in his eyes and fingers that indicate, to them, that he can hear them. In fact they are convinced that he can now give them a thumbs-up sign. Indeed, in November 2012, even to the doctors, he did appear to "lighten" a little in his unresponsive state, and so his condition was upgraded to a "minimally conscious state." Hassan's doctors thought he might, sometimes, be able to receive and respond to *some* stimuli on *some* level. But was this an improvement in Hassan's condition?

The diagnosis of patients in these states is sometimes backed up by further testing, such as by EEGs, brain circulation studies, and, more recently, a functional MRI, which attempts to correlate cerebral responses with blood flow. The fMRI is still considered experimental, but Sunnybrook offered to bring in an outside expert to carry out this test on Hassan in order to more objectively determine his actual level of awareness. Hassan's family grasped at this opportunity, but the results were equivocal. Even this ambiguous outcome, however, provided some hope for the family.

During our meeting, Parichehr unfolded a newspaper article describing how an Alfred Hitchcock movie presented to some patients in a persistent vegetative state elicited, in fMRI recordings, a brain response similar to that seen in normal patients. The significance of these findings is disputed in the medical community. Do these patients truly respond on some cognitive or emotional or sentient level? Are such patients "locked in" there, somewhere?

"The doctors were wrong to say 'permanent,'" Parichehr told me. "Maybe he will recover even more." Patients in a minimally conscious state are almost never as they were before their comatose condition. They remain profoundly impaired neurologically. But Hassan *had* recrossed the line.

What would the optimal setting and stimulation be for such a patient? Hassan's family hopes he will improve more with brain stimulation, something that is hard to provide in an acute care hospital. It is also something that is controversial. The family hoped Hassan would be transferred to a rehabilitation institution where he might receive a different kind of care. But there are too few institutions with the capacity to accept such ventilator-dependent, debilitated patients.

The medical profession views efforts to maintain or improve the condition of these persistently comatose patients as, ultimately, futile. To doctors, such patients are almost dead already. What the family saw as responsiveness in Hassan, the doctors saw as primitive reflex reactions. What the family interpreted as evidence of Hassan's being awake, they took to be the random cycle of yawning and eyes opening that occurs in patients in a vegetative state. Movements of his eyes were not tracking motion but were random actions.

The argument is made that, if unawareness is permanent, as it is taken to be in a *permanent* vegetative state, then the patient can never experience any benefit, so any treatment provided should be for comfort care only.

Yet even this notion of "comfort" is questionable, for such patients would not experience any suffering in being allowed to die. The physicians argue that it is not within the standard of care (the usual treatment) to indefinitely support someone who will *never* recover. There is no person there to nurture and protect. So, treat them with basic, respectful nursing care, yes, but anything more aggressive, no. If a serious infection, organ failure, or cardiac or respiratory arrest occurs, it is best to let death happen.

By current medical standards, patients in persistent or permanent vegetative states are considered irrecoverably lost. They might be "in there" in some way, but where and how to reach them remain unknown. As with sailors lost at sea, we spend only so long looking for them. The problem in Hassan's case is that he *had* recovered somewhat—he is in a minimally conscious state. Nevertheless, the prognosis for patients in this state, although largely unexplored, is thought to be little better than for those in a vegetative state.

Perhaps this is the quality of mercy in our health care system. Merciful treatment is rarely bestowed indefinitely. How, it may be asked, can we justify spending weeks, months, or even years, and millions of dollars, looking for one lost sailor—or one deeply comatose patient? The problem is we don't know when to say no, when to say enough is enough. Our knowledge is imperfect, our resources are finite, and our dominant values and preferences are various and change—that is why, in part, when doctors try to say no to some patients, we are hesitant and inconsistent. Why can some get expensive high-tech care while others get little at all? We have an obligation to preserve life, but there is also an acknowledgement everywhere that humans at times need to recognize the limits to care and allow nature to take its course.

How much better it would be if we knew there were certain states in which each patient would not want to be kept alive, if hospitals asked patients, especially patients facing major surgery, clear and pointed questions in advance: If you were in a non-responsive or minimally responsive state, how would you want to be treated? If you also had only the remotest prospect of even partial recovery, would you wish to be kept going by expensive and prolonged measures? And what if, on account of that care, others were deprived of truly effective care? Would you still want be kept alive?

Hospitals and health professionals in Canada too rarely ask patients about such matters. They ought to and are encouraged to do so. But if they don't, patients and their families *must* consider these tough questions themselves.

"Death is a mercy," people sometimes say. Even if patients lingering in a persistent vegetative state or in a minimally conscious state may not be suffering physically, they could be experiencing profound and deep psychological distress. What is left intact will vary from one patient to the next. What the person may be experiencing, if anything, is currently unknown. Living in this state could be like living in a fragmentary dream-like state, the equivalent of being buried alive. One prominent philosopher has written of "the terrifying state of those who have lost any sense of their own self, and cannot seize on any self to think of."[3] Life then would consist of fragmentary bits of sensory data with fear and pain being experienced by, but inexplicable to, the patient. The thread of life would be lost, for no central, unifying sense of self would be present.

Shortly after Hassan was diagnosed as being in a persistent vegetative state, his family was told, they say, that the clinicians were entitled to decide on their own to stop life-supporting treatment and that they would do so, and that Parichehr, as Hassan's substitute decision maker, would need a court order if she wished to carry on with treatment. At least that is what the family understood. But Parichehr and her children were determined not to be moved.

Once the conflict between the family and Hassan's doctors was revealed, and when it became absolutely clear that the family would not consent to the withdrawal of life support as the doctors had advised, there was, under Ontario's Health Care Consent Act, a legislated avenue for resolving the conflict. Hassan's doctors might have sought direction from a quasi-judicial tribunal devoted to resolving disputes over care. Ontario's Consent and Capacity

Board, consisting most often of three individuals—a doctor, a lawyer, and a member of the public—is meant to provide a neutral oversight for capacity assessments, treatment decisions, and some, but *only some*, end-of-life disputes. The board has a clear role when it comes to decisions over the appropriate *provision* of care; it has been less clear that its mandate extends to the *non*-provision of care.

In any case, Hassan's doctors did not want to go before the board. Hassan's life was too irrevocably degraded to warrant indefinite intensive care treatment. He would never experience any benefit from life-sustaining interventions such as artificial nutrition and machine-assisted breathing support. The doctors believed that to keep these measures going for Hassan, after he had spent three years in an unaware state, was futile for the patient, harmful to others (who may as a result not have had access to limited equipment or resources), and contrary to professional medical standards of care.

This was a point of principle for them as physicians as well as a point of legal clarity. Should the board decide in favour of the family, how could the physicians in good conscience prescribe or continue a treatment that they saw as ineffectual? To suggest that they ignore their own views in such cases would be asking them to suspend their professional training and obligations. Is a surgeon expected to perform surgery on an unsuitable candidate? So, they would argue, what role could or should an external tribunal play in deciding about the efficacy of care?

For the doctors it was a question of the standard of care and who should define it.

Hassan's family had little objective medical evidence on which to base their requests for further intensive care. Through her lawyers, Parichehr did file the medical assessments of Hassan's shifting diagnosis from a persistent vegetative state to a minimally conscious state. But doubts about the quality of his life remained. To establish Hassan's wishes, Parichehr cited his religious faith—as a devout Shia Muslim—as proof that he would want to be kept alive in these circumstances, until there were no signs of life. She remained unshakable in her belief that Hassan would want his life to be preserved no matter how poor its quality might be. Hassan may have had a certain commitment to life at any cost, but would it have encompassed *this* type of life and for *this* long a period? His family is firmly convinced it would.

This desire to continue Hassan's life in his present state is not dependent on a religious view of life. Needless suffering is not a virtue in any religion. The acknowledgement of the limits of human powers at life's end is present in all religions, including Islam. Wanting to keep Hassan going is, rather, a result of a set of secular and very modern beliefs that puts stock in what *science* has done, is doing, and will do for Hassan. Death, with science's help, becomes a negotiated event that can be postponed indefinitely.

Hassan Rasouli's case went all the way to the Supreme Court of Canada. It ruled in a 5–2 decision that the physicians could not, without the consent of Hassan's family, stop his treatment. The majority judgment acknowledged the doctors' assessment of their patient's situation—that life support conferred no medical benefit for him—and noted that this opinion appeared to reflect a widely accepted view in the medical community. The judges, however, based their ruling on a statutory interpretation of Ontario's Health Care Consent Act. They argued that if Hassan's ventilator stopped, the doctors would have to provide palliative care. The cessation of one treatment would require the starting of *another*, for which consent would be needed. It was for *this* step that the doctors would require the consent of Hassan's substitute decision maker. And this was precisely what Parichehr refused to accept.

It was the *doctors*, not Parichehr, who would need a court order to stop treatment. If the physicians could not come to an agreement with the family, the court said, then they should take the case to the Consent and Capacity Board.

The case has stopped there. The physicians have not gone to the Board, perhaps reasoning that they have expended enough energy already and perhaps reckoning that there may be some uncertainty about the acceptability of their opposition to treatment given that Hassan is in a minimally conscious state, and his prognosis is therefore a *little* less certain than if he had remained in a vegetative state. I understand that his profoundly debilitated state continues.

The court's ruling seemed to be a watershed victory for patients and families over doctors. But Hassan's family hardly experienced it as a victory.

How families and patients can and should work together with health professionals—especially across cultural divides—is always a challenge. But a realistic (as opposed to wishful) appreciation of what is important for life and what medicine can do for patients is essential. Wishes alone cannot and should not always dictate care.

I doubt there was anything the hospital or the doctors involved could have done to prevent this impasse, once Hassan was comatose. Had, however, there been an explicit discussion with Hassan before his brain surgery about his wishes if his medical care went awry, it is quite possible that he, like most people, would have declined intensive care should his brain be as injured as it was. There is some debate about which patients should have their preferences for life-sustaining care elicited in advance, but one circumstance would surely be anyone undergoing brain surgery.

This is an area that has dramatically changed over the thirty-five years since I started my medical training. That patients should have a full say in and control over their health care is a modern idea that has transformed medical practice. Patients have the right to make treatment decisions in advance in case they should lose their ability to make their wishes clear. Patients also have the right to reject any treatment at all—no matter how beneficial it is, even if life-saving. It would be considered substandard care for a physician not to know a patient's wishes in this regard, if the patient is known to them.

Parichehr and her children were tenacious in their advocacy for Hassan. They showed that families could resist what physicians wanted and considered reasonable—that David could defeat a modern Goliath. But their situation—and Hassan's—is not an enviable one. His is not a state from which meaningful recovery will ever be possible. Neither side wins in the contested battle over the disposition of the patient who remains so ill, living in a netherworld of consciousness.

SUFFER THE CHILDREN

Christine Ho was a good girl. The only child of immigrant parents from Hong Kong who looked to her as their future, she was expected to do well in school, and she did. Christine was quiet. Several times during her clinic visits to me, I would have to ask her to speak up, and my efforts at small talk were never very successful. One of Christine's parents, usually her father, would accompany her to these appointments. He was a stern man. I don't recall ever seeing him smile. On her tenth birthday, Christine came in with her unsmiling father for her annual physical. I took her blood pressure, noted her height and weight.

Christine was particularly taciturn that day. I asked her to lie down on the examination table. She did so, but when I went to do an abdominal exam she said, "No!"

and wouldn't let me touch her. I tried to make a joke of it, but she wouldn't relent. I had been seeing Christine since she was quite small, and somehow it had escaped me that she was on the cusp of adolescence. I had not only failed to ask her father to leave the examining room; I had asked him to give me a hand. I needed to examine Christine's abdomen as part of the physical, but what little history I could get from her—that she threw up sometimes and had little appetite—made me worried enough that I thought her abdomen *should* be examined.

Once her father was involved, a struggle of wills ensued: her resistance to the examination and my obstinate desire to continue. Of course, two men against one child—she had to give in. And, much to my surprise, and her father's, I found a small mass in her abdomen. I wondered if she had been in pain, and for how long. Had she told anyone about the pain—her parents, a teacher, a friend—and if not, why? I never had the chance to ask, though. It seems my treatment of Christine had caused a rift in our relationship. She would need further tests, such as an ultrasound, which I ordered, but before the tests were completed, the family asked a colleague of mine to take over Christine's care.

It turned out that the mass I palpated was her spleen, enlarged because of a lymphoma. Christine's cancer was caught early, and luckily it was very responsive to treatment.

What continued to bother me, though, was the examination we had forced on Christine. Although some good came of it, I am not sure I was justified in my insistence that she be examined there and then. Christine could have come back another day, when she felt more comfortable. Before the examination began, I could have—I *should* have—asked Christine's father to leave and the female clinic nurse to join me. Perhaps that would have been less threatening. Examining a resisting child had felt like an assault on Christine's dignity and on her bodily integrity, too. But later, as I considered the situation, I thought, *What if I hadn't found the mass that day? I might not have seen her for another year. And by then it may have been too late.*

Every day, physicians must weigh the risks of intervening, to try to prevent avoidable harms to a resistant patient, against not intervening. The answer depends, in large measure, on the mental capacity of the patient. Who has the right to say no to an examination, a test, a treatment? Does this right extend to minors? Some people argue that children are too limited in their experience to make medical decisions and that what is needed is their "assent" to treatment, that their agreement to go along with treatment—or an examination—should be sought in any way possible.

These issues rose to prominence in Canada with the life and death of young Makayla Sault. Makayla's case raised complex questions not only about the capacity needed to consent, or not, to treatment, but also about the influence of culture in medical decision making. My views about Makayla's withdrawal from conventional care have changed over time. At first I was sure this was a clear case of child mistreatment or abandonment. Later, I was not so sure.[1]

Makayla Sault said Jesus visited her in a dream. Makayla was an eleven-year-old member of the Mississaugas of the New Credit First Nation in southern Ontario. She had been diagnosed with an aggressive form of acute lympho blastic leukemia, a cancer of the blood cells in her bone marrow, and had undergone a very unpleasant eleven-week in-hospital course of chemotherapy in 2014. During her hospitalization, she became nauseated, shed her hair, lost weight, and lost all her energy. Her reaction to the treatment was so severe that she was moved to the intensive care unit at McMaster Children's Hospital.

Makayla said she knew her visitor was Jesus because he showed her his hands and they had holes in them. He was accompanied by two large angels and was dressed in a white robe with a purple sash. She said he had shoulder-length straight brown hair. Makayla thought he looked beautiful. Jesus told her that she was already cured. She knew then that it was time to stop her treatment and stay off it.

Makayla wanted to be at home. Her parents, both pastors at a local church, supported Makayla in her refusal of treatment. Makayla had always been a mature child and was involved in all the decisions concerning her recent medical care. They were not about to overrule her. But now she was leaving the hospital against firm medical advice. This was an unusual decision for the team looking after her, as it meant undermining the only chance she had of a more permanent regression of her blood disorder. The chemotherapy she had already had was only an introduction to treatment; she would require many more rounds of chemotherapy and perhaps stem cell or bone marrow replacements. A few weeks after the chemo was stopped and she was back at home, Makayla said she was eating and feeling better. Her mother would say later that, after Makayla left the hospital, she continued to receive treatment from her family physician. As well, she continued to see an oncologist at the McMaster Children's Hospital. She had also started to receive a traditional medicine from a healer near her home. Though this traditional medicine is untested by science, its effectiveness is supported by a long and strong oral history, and it has apparently helped others in Makayla's community.

In a letter Makayla wrote to her doctors, and which she read on a video produced by *Two Row Times*, a free newspaper serving the Six Nations, she explained, "Jesus came into my room, and he told me not to be afraid, so if I live or if I die, I am not afraid."[2] She begged her parents not to send her back to hospital. She wanted to go off chemo, she said, as it was "killing" her.

To outsiders, it would seem unlikely that Makayla would have had the capacity to make a life-and-death decision. In many jurisdictions, children below a certain age—fourteen in Quebec, sixteen in many American states, eighteen in others—do not have the authority to make serious medical decisions. These age limits in law appear to acknowledge the emotional and cognitive immaturity of most children. But all children are not the same. At a very early age some master, for example, the intense complexities of playing a musical instrument. Some have high emotional IQs, and others can understand the abstractions of calculus. To some children, developmentally sophisticated skills come early and are exercised with a maturity far beyond their years.

So the real sticking point for many people was Makayla's age. An eleven-year-old being allowed to refuse chemo? *Really?*

In some modernized countries the medico-legal world slowly started to come around to the decision-making rights of children in the 1970s and 1980s. In 1985, in the U.K., Victoria Gillick, a mother of five young daughters, found out that local health authorities would, if requested, prescribe the birth control pill to girls under sixteen without their parents' knowledge. Mrs. Gillick went to court over this. She did not want her daughters to have access to the pill without her being informed.

After a series of appeals, the House of Lords ruled against her. It observed that parents' authority over their children "dwindled" as they grew older, as their children's capacity for understanding increased.[3] In the U.K., then, "mature" children—determined not by age but by their mental capacity—could get a prescription for birth control without their parents ever being involved.

This was a limited victory for children's rights. If a teen were to refuse *life-sustaining* medical treatment, in the U.K.—and in many other places as well—consent can be sought from a parent or someone else responsible for the child's welfare.[4] Children are considered capable of seeking life-changing, albeit less momentous, medical treatments such as birth control, but not considered so wise as to make life-and-death decisions for themselves.

However, the view that children *could* be capable of making important decisions concerning their lives, including refusing life-sustaining care, found some favour in North America. Under Ontario's Health Care Consent Act, passed in 1996, for example, there is no fixed age of consent—everything depends on the child's mental capacity to understand and appreciate the requisite information. Capacity is never an all-or-nothing concept—the child's capacity may fluctuate, and the ability to give consent may depend on the gravity and complexity of the decision to be made.[5] What is in a child's best interests must take into account not only what *medicine* deems to be the best but also what the *child* thinks as well.

This more tolerant view of a child's capacity distinguishes a child's ability to understand and appreciate the consequences for *themselves* as opposed to the more extensive and abstract mental skills required to make decisions for others. It is not chronological age but, rather, experience that is the most salient factor in determining whether a child is sufficiently mature to make medical decisions.[6]

In her study of British children, some as young as eight, undergoing serious orthopaedic surgery (including amputations and bone cancer surgery), Priscilla Alderson observed that "small, immature bodies are generally believed to contain small, immature minds." She noted that the researchers "had not anticipated the amount of suffering the children were expected to accept—or consent to."[7]

If we expect children to suffer, do we not have an obligation to involve them as much as possible, and as much as they want to be involved, in important decisions concerning their lives? If we agree that we do, then it was especially important to seek Makayla's authorization for the treatment being administered to her.

One mark of immaturity is an inability to see forward—to make decisions that delay gratification and that may involve short-term pain for long-term gain. This is why most children will, if given the choice, turn down immunization or ill-tasting medication. *They don't know what is good for them*, we say.

This psychological characteristic did not, however—at least as seen from a distance, anyway—appear to apply to Makayla. What was astonishing in this case was the maturity and calmness with which Makayla faced her situation. Makayla said she knew she could die without further chemotherapy. She understood this to be Jesus's plan for her. There was a clear religious element to her decision, but this is hardly unusual and does not make her decision either irrational or unworthy of respect. It does require investigation, however, to ensure she was not under the undue influence of others.

The standard response, well articulated by North American and English courts since the 1920s, is that parents can make martyrs of themselves for the sake of their religion, but they may not make martyrs of their children. Only when they are considered capable or mature may children make judgments that go contrary to their medically determined best interests, especially when it comes to life-and-death decisions. This is a reasonable compromise between self-determination and the duty to rescue.

If Makayla had been considered incapable of making mature decisions about her own care, and her parents were viewed as not promoting her best interests, the child welfare authorities could have stepped in. When Makayla refused further chemotherapy, the McMaster Children's Hospital asked Brant Family and Children's Services to investigate the case. The agency did so, but it did *not* apprehend Makayla, something for which it was roundly criticized by the press and the health care community.

In May 2014, weeks after Makayla decided to stop chemotherapy treatment, the agency closed her file. "We feel that Makayla is in a loving, caring home and that they are carrying on with medicine that would be very appropriate for a First Nations family," explained executive director Andrew Koster. McMaster also issued a statement, saying the hospital respected the society's decision and felt for the "heartbreaking circumstance" the Sault family was in. "It is the role of the Children's Aid Society to weigh circumstances and make the difficult decisions they do about protecting children and preserving families," the statement read. "It is our role at McMaster Children's Hospital to provide the best possible care for children, using the best medical evidence."

Serious arguments backed up by good reasons were raised from differing viewpoints when Makayla's refusal of treatment, and the failure of the child welfare authorities to even try to authorize treatment for her, became public knowledge. Some people (especially from her community) supported Makayla's right to choose her own treatment.[8] What was originally an issue between the child and her parents and some of the health care professionals in Hamilton escalated into a political debate about the historical treatment of indigenous people in Canada. "We're never going to allow another agency to ever do that to us again, where they remove our children from their community, from their culture, from their traditions," said Chief Bryan LaForme of the New Credit First Nation. Recalling the long history of injustice—of native children being taken from their families and forced into the harsh environment of residential schools—the leader concluded, "We are not going to let foreign governments come in and apprehend children."[9]

Makayla's mother has said that before referring the case to the children's aid society, the hospital threatened to have the authorities apprehend Makayla so that treatment could be forced upon her. A defence force was set up around Makayla and her family to prevent the authorities from abducting her. Makayla's parents and her community thus had both immediate and historical reasons to feel protective.

Beyond her community, many were impressed by Makayla's maturity and determination. Supporters of her choice emphasized the potential toxicity and the debilitating side effects of chemotherapy. Others pointed to the very high success rate of chemotherapy as a treatment for children with the same form of leukemia as Makayla's, and to the 100 per cent certainty of the cancer's recurrence without treatment.

Makayla's parents said they were worried that the toxicity of chemotherapy would not be balanced by its benefits. How certain was it that chemotherapy would help Makayla? On the one hand, the treatment of childhood acute lymphoblastic leukemia is one of modern medicine's success stories. In 1960, children with the disease were given no chance of surival. Now, with chemotherary and bone marrow transplantation the five-year survival has reached 90 per cent. On the other hand, 80 per cent of children will experience a serious or even life-threatening complication from the intensified treatments now used. Makayla's leukemia was Philadelphia chromosome-positive, a factor that reduced her five-year survival rate to 70 percent.

The required treatment for Makayla's cancer is an uncertain enterprise, and some regimens, such as the chemotherapy, can be extremely taxing and require assiduous patient compliance for extended periods. The idea of imposing such treatment on a resisting child is a distressing one to contemplate. Would they tie her down for the many intravenous treatments she would require? The *consequences* of enforced treatment for Makayla—both physically and to her dignity as a human being—would, almost certainly, have been much worse than the consequences of a forced examination were for my patient Christine.

To many outside observers at the time, myself included, things seemed to be simple ethically: this was just a rerun of the problem of Jehovah's Witness parents refusing life-sustaining blood products for their child.[10] In such a situation, the parents' views are nullified by the needs of their dependent children.

I now think, however, that this model—having the state step in to make decisions for ill children that their parents should have made—may be the wrong one to use in Makayla's case. The law authorizes intervention in emergency situations, such as when a child is bleeding to death and there is no time to assess his or her mental capacity. A one-time intervention in an emergency is one thing, but a more extensive regimen of somewhat uncertain treatments over months and maybe years is another.

Makayla seemed to know full well what the consequences of refusing treatment might be. She was not in as urgent need of being rescued as a child who is bleeding to death and whose parents are refusing to authorize a blood transfusion for her. She appeared to be mature, thoughtful, and worldly-wise. And, unlike most of us, she had experience of chemotherapy. Together these are, ultimately, the *only* good reasons for which she could have been allowed to refuse care. If there were no uncertainties in her resolve or her capacity and all options for treatment had been exhausted (or they were all equally burdensome), then the decision to respect Makayla's wish not to receive chemotherapy was the appropriate one. Less than a year after she refused conventional treatment, Makayla's immune system failed and she died of an overwhelming infection and a cerebral stroke. Her family attributes her death to the chemotherapy she received.[11] Needless to say, this was disputed by health care authorities, who attributed her death to her untreated leukemia.

Just how to achieve compromise and accommodation with families, and how far to pursue resistant child-age patients or their families, depends on the circumstances: How urgent is the problem? How serious is it? How entrenched is the family in their views? What are the chances of success of treatment? These questions may be difficult to answer with certainty, which is one more reason to urge caution and restraint. While such questions cannot deter health professionals from trying to rescue critically ill patients, deference must be given to families who care for their children and disagree about the likelihood of the success of treatments. It is not just children from indigenous communities who may be allowed to refuse potentially life-sustaining treatment.

In other places and at other times, parents have been allowed to refuse life-sustaining treatment for their children. For example, in 1991 a Saskatchewan couple was allowed to refuse a liver transplant for their infant daughter who was dying of biliary atresia, a condition that is fatal without a transplant and carries a 65 per cent five-year chance of survival with one. The judge in that case remarked that the parents acted in the "caring and thoughtful way" society expects parents to behave.[12] This is very similar to the situation in which Makayla and her family found themselves. We have to accept the possibility, indeed the probability, that at times there are many differences—not just cultural and familial—that may constitute good and justifiable reasons for capable patients and families to act in ways that the mainstream culture will find unacceptable.

Thus, Makayla's situation is not unique. Treating any child with a serious disorder, like cancer, diabetes, or anorexia nervosa, conditions that require continuing and serious interventions, calls for special care. Health care professionals must work *with* their patients, not against them. This requires an inclusive approach to treatment planning as well as respect for deeply held values and views.

In general, providing an opening for compromise and listening to the concerns of patients and families is the best action to take. It is critical for health professionals to work cooperatively with families, especially across cultural divides, to tell them from the outset what to look out for, to explain the potential effects of treatments. When medical teams are open and transparent, patients and their families are more likely to develop trust in them and less likely to be swayed primarily, or solely, by limited cultural influences. Of course, another way to navigate cultural divides in such situations is to promote the medical training of members of the cultural tradition in question, so that the cultural divisions may be bridged, not eliminated.[13] This has only recently started to happen in Canada.

Working in a harmonious and collaborative way with families—trying to derive a treatment plan that respects or reflects their perspectives—is the way for health care professionals to proceed. If families and children adamantly refuse life-saving treatment, one should at least attempt to ensure clinical vigilance. Makayla was followed regularly, though it did not suffice to prevent her death.

In the fall of 2014, there was a new case of a child with the same kind of cancer as Makayla's. J.J. was an eleven-year-old girl from the Iroquois Six Nations Reserve near where Makayla lived. Her mother, acting as her substitute decision maker, had rejected chemotherapy on her behalf and removed her from the hospital after less than two weeks of treatment.[14] The hospital immediately contacted Brant Family and Children's Services, seeking its intervention to bring J.J. back into chemotherapy treatment as soon as possible. When the agency decided not to intervene, Hamilton Health Sciences Corporation made an application under Ontario's Child and Family Services Act to have her named a child in need of protection.[15] There was clear evidence offered before the court in Brantford, Ontario, that J.J. was, unlike Makayla, incapable and that it was her mother who was making the decision not to allow chemotherapy. Trying to exercise a Solomon-like wisdom, Mr. Justice Gethin Edward found that J.J., although having a terrible disease, was not a child in need of protection. Rather, she was being cared for according to beliefs and practices that were central to, and constitutive of, an aboriginal community. All parties agreed that her mother was a devoted parent, trying to do the best for J.J. The judgment is a thoughtful consideration of the issues at stake and is a challenge to reasoning that focuses narrowly on autonomy and beneficence. What is in a patient's best interests is intimately connected with her views and wishes, expressed in J.J.'s case by her mother. But another factor that should be considered is the principle of justice or fairness. One way of considering this is to ask: Was J.J. receiving care that would be considered reasonable by her community at large?

Touching upon this question, Justice Edward reminded all involved in J.J.'s case of the reason aboriginal rights exist at all. He quoted Supreme Court Chief Justice Antonio Lamer, who wrote, "When Europeans arrived in North America, aboriginal peoples *were already here*, living in . . . distinctive cultures, as they had done for centuries. It is this fact . . . which separates aboriginal peoples from all other minority groups in Canadian society." Lamer went on to explain that an aboriginal right to be protected by law "must be an element of a practice, custom or tradition integral to the distinctive culture of the aboriginal group claiming the right . . . A practical way of thinking about this problem is to ask whether, without this practice, tradition or custom, the culture in question would be fundamentally altered or other than what it is."

Justice Edward found there was good evidence that traditional medicine was integral to the Six Nations community. The commitment of J.J.'s mother to this tradition was not, in his words, "an eleventh-hour epiphany employed to take her daughter out of the rigors of che-motherapy." Her decision to pursue traditional therapy was her aboriginal right. This right "cannot be qualified as a right only if it [the traditional therapy] is proven to work by employing the western medical paradigm. To do so would be to leave open the opportunity to perpet-ually erode aboriginal rights." Hence, he dismissed the hospital's application that J.J. be declared a child in need of protection. She was being cared for, and so ostensibly protected, by a different set of beliefs.

But was there not a certain skepticism about "Western" science and medicine that was unspoken in this judgment? How else could the judge conceive that one approach might be as good as the other? The judg-ment simply appears to suggest that our knowledge—anyone's set of beliefs or practices—is always limited in scope and dependability. Contemporary medicine is itself hardly a monolithic enterprise and is constantly being revised. There are always conflicts in society over the best way to live. Justice Edward was not prepared to say that indigenous practices about health were so outlandish as to exclude their consideration as a defensible and just way of caring for a sick child. When J.J.'s leukemia recurred in March 2015, she restarted chemotherapy while continu-ing with traditional medicine.

Known for his novel approaches to the people and cases he rules on, Justice Edward, after prompting by the Ministry of the Attorney General, clarified the reasons for his judgment in the case of J.J. "It does no mischief to my decision to recognize that the best interests of the child remain paramount," he said in May 2015.[16] To some, this may seem like trying to fit a square peg into a round hole. *Either* the child's interests are paramount *or* the culture's interests are. But to others it simply recommends that one should consider *both* sides of a position before taking a stand on principle. Stands on principles alone— either by patients, their families, or health care professionals—may be brave, but they can also be unnecessarily dangerous and may prevent examination of the nuances and details of a situation. Better to strive towards a perspective-less view of ethics by trying to work with and combine different beliefs and convictions. Ethics does not belong to one culture or community. It tries to express a view that all could and should respect.

This judgment, then, suggests a step away from cultural relativism and a way out of the impasse in cases such as this. First and foremost, we must avoid either-or-ism and try to find common ground. Health care professionals need to try to understand the patient's and the family's distinct perspectives. Authentic aboriginal cultural and medicinal traditions should not be dismissed out of hand. Complementary approaches are needed.[17]

Secondly, patients and their families need to try to recognize what modern medicine may offer in the way of curative therapies. When a child's welfare is at stake, finding ways to compromise and work together—by combining the best of traditional medicine with the best that modern medicine can offer—is the best approach.

Thirdly, there is no one way to be an "authentic" member of a community. Cultures are always riven by conflicts between the orthodox and all the others. Despite having the same culture or heritage, people will choose very differently for a variety of personal, religious, and familial reasons. The challenge is to enable them to make the decisions that are right for them.

Trying to respect wishes while protecting a patient's best interests is a struggle not without precedent. Although it can be particularly tragic when it involves the care of children, the conflict plays out in end-of-life care for adults, too.

VIII

QUITTING TIME

Afterwards, in the ICU, Katie Aronowitz told me how scared she had been. It was the late fall of 2000, and Katie had gone to the house of her grandfather, Sam Artinian, for a visit. When he didn't answer the door, she let herself in, and found Sam in his bed. Katie was frightened—at first glance she thought he was dead, and she was unable to rouse him. Only while gently shaking him did she realize he was *not* dead—he was feverish and pink. She dialed 911.

Sam, his wife, and members of his extended family had been my patients for years. He was a handsome, cultivated man, debonair, always polite, always well dressed. Sam was in "good enough" health for someone in his mid-eighties—intact cognitively, no heart disease, no diabetes, just some mild hypertension. Not all was well with him, however. His wife had advanced dementia and did not recognize him when he visited her in the nursing home where she had resided for the last few years. And Sam's strength was gradually failing him. He had been unable to keep up his much-loved country farm where, more for fun than profit, he raised Christmas trees, and he had to sell it.

Sam's family knew he'd been unhappy for some time. He felt that his best years were behind him. "What's the use of going on? I've lived long enough," he would say to his family, his friends, to me, to anyone who'd listen. "No heroics for me. Please, just let me go."

A month before Katie found him in his bed, Sam had been in my office, and for some reason we had a conversation about his views on end-of-life care.

"What if your illness is treatable?" I asked him. "Say you were seriously ill with an infection and needed intensive care for a brief period?" In many people's minds, a temporary period of dependence on technology is different from permanently being hooked up to machines with tubes in every orifice. "Would you accept life support if it was only temporary?"

"No way. You doctors say 'temporary,' and before you know it, it's weeks later and the patient is still hooked up to the breathing machine. Nope. I don't want any of it!"

"Would you not be giving up too readily?"

"Look, Doctor, I know you're doing your best, but really, my answer is still no. I've had a good life. Let me go when I get sick. Please."

"What about your family? Have you considered them?"

"My family doesn't need me to be around. I don't want to be a burden and be unable to look after myself."

I knew Sam had been seeing a psychiatrist for depression, and I asked him if depression might be influencing his position on treatment.

Sam laughed. "Come on now. Do I look depressed to you? I am tired and fed up. My family knows how I feel. I'm being realistic. What do I have to look forward to? Having some illness like my wife's? Being institutionalized and fed by someone else's hand? Soiling my underwear and having someone else wipe my butt? The idea of this is more than I can bear. No, thank you! When my time comes, just let me go, okay? As I said, no heroics." Sam grew animated. "I hope you're writing all this down! I don't want to have to repeat myself." It wasn't just a conversation; he was giving me instructions.

It sounded to me as if Sam would welcome a sudden death. And it sounded as if he wanted it to come soon. Although his psychiatrist would later attest to Sam's dissatisfaction with life, there was no evidence that he was actively considering suicide. And there was nothing, he would say later (and I would concur), to suggest that Sam even needed medication for depression.

In the ER that day, the cause of Sam's state was not obvious. He still couldn't be roused. (He was obtunded, as we say in medicine.) He was not breathing well enough on his own, so he was intubated. He was then transferred to the ICU. His diagnosis was respiratory failure NYD, meaning not yet diagnosed. Blood samples were taken, a lumbar puncture was done, and X-rays ordered. The results of all these tests were normal—no stroke, no heart attack, no sepsis, no drugs, no obvious malignancy, and no evidence of attempted suicide. In short, no answers.

The next day, while Sam was still unconscious, one of his daughters, Lilly Aronowitz, Katie's mother, arrived from out of town. Lilly was not pleased that her father had been put on a ventilator. She knew he would not have wanted it. She affirmed that her sisters would agree with her.

Lilly watched her father's chest rise and fall with each piston-like hiss of the ventilator. She asked the nurse looking after Sam if his treatment could be stopped. Hard to do that now, she was told, since they didn't know what happened to her father. Maybe he would recover. Time sometimes makes all things clear.

Lilly was upset. "How long will he be in the ICU?" she asked the ICU resident. "What more tests do you need to do? And how sure are you that you'll find out what's wrong with my father?" The resident wasn't entirely sure of the answers. Even in the best of circumstances, Lilly's questions would not all be readily answerable. ICU care is rarely simple or straightforward.

"He wouldn't want this, you know," Lilly said to me when we met in the ICU. Her two siblings, who had arrived at the hospital, agreed. I had come to see Sam in a dual role—as his family physician and as the ethics consultant. I felt his daughters were almost certainly right, but there were still many unknowns in Sam's case. I suggested it might be better to wait another day or two for more answers before withdrawing care.

But after three days in the ICU there was still no clear diagnosis other than coma due to respiratory failure, or coma causing respiratory decline. Which was cause and which effect was unknown—and maybe unknowable. More investigations and more time, perhaps days or weeks even, would be required. In the meantime Sam would have to be kept on life support, something he had said to me quite strenuously that he would not want, even temporarily. We were ignoring his marching orders.

From the ICU perspective, no patient is considered hopeless until all the stones have been turned over. Sam was not, as yet, hopeless. Doctors, who work with mysterious, enigmatic conditions all the time, are used to the rigours of the ICU. Patients and families are not.

I was somewhat conflicted in my two roles. As his family doctor I did not want to lose Sam. But it is not the role of the ethics consultant to tell the people involved what to do. It is to uncover the values involved in a case, to explore with families and health care professionals the possible options, and to try to ensure that the "right" thing is done. The ethics consultant may sometimes be seen as a *guarantor* of right outcomes, but he or she is not.

The ethicist is more akin to the ancient poet Virgil, who accompanied Dante on his descent into the Inferno: making him aware of the dangers, introducing him to the right people, learning the haunting stories of others.

Despite the mystery surrounding Sam's illness, there was a convergence of opinion regarding his care. Input from those who knew him—from his psychiatrist, myself, and his daughters—indicated that the longer aggressive care was continued, the more his wishes were being ignored. There was no evidence that Sam was suffering from a major depression or had tried to end his life. Sam would not thank his family or the medical team, even if he could be saved. I imagined the conversation I would have with him if he survived but faced months of rehabilitation: *Why didn't you just let me go? Now look at me! What good am I to anyone—especially to myself?* He would have had no heart for the hard work rehab would require. Like the tortured souls awoken by Dante's intrusion into their territory, who clamoured to return to sleep, Sam would not have been happy with a continued life. It would have been a torture for him.

So, when Sam didn't rouse even a little by the fifth day in ICU, the medical team agreed that he should be removed from the ventilator. If he rallied and breathed on his own, that was fine. However, the likelihood of that happening was considered vanishingly small.

Lilly, her two siblings, and Katie gathered around Sam's bed, watching as the ICU resident carefully and quickly removed his breathing tube. After several minutes his breathing slowed down and his pulse stopped. I told his weeping family that he had passed away.

However, I had spoken too soon. Sam took a deep breath and kept on breathing for a few minutes more, albeit in a gradually diminishing way. He then stopped breathing altogether. When his pulse ceased, the resident pronounced that Sam was dead.

It may seem that the way things turned out with Sam was not that challenging. But in fact it was. While the evidence from those who knew Sam pointed in one direction—that it was time to let him go—not everyone was so sure that the decision to remove Sam from life support was the right thing to do. For his health care providers, the nagging worry was that they might still have found a reversible cause for Sam's decline.

Moreover, just because in the end we all agreed on a course of action does not mean it was the right or only one to take. Were we guilty of groupthink, a recognized hazard of team decision making in which the desire for consensus overrides common sense? I do not, in retrospect, think so. The medical team had listened carefully and closely to what Sam's family was telling us. We entertained all views. We considered everything about Sam's prospects, in the light of what was known at the time, as limited as that might have been. The ideal in ethics is to try to attain the *perspective-less* view, but this can, paradoxically, only be achieved by looking at the situation from different perspectives. The most challenging situations are those in which health care professionals are faced with conflicting and unyielding opinions about what the patient would have wanted.

It was April 2004, and Ralph Fields had had a terrible week. On Monday his wife, Elaine, had wandered from home. The police found her several blocks away, in her nightgown and in an agitated state, and took her back home.

This wasn't the first time Elaine had wandered. This time she had managed to escape while Ralph was on the phone. When police brought her home she was confused. Ralph and his wife had moved to a smaller house two years before, when Elaine's memory was starting to fail. Apparently, she had never become used to their new home and thought she belonged back at their old address. Ralph reassured the police that they were all right, double-locking the doors as they left.

Wandering wasn't Elaine's only problem. She had had progressive memory loss for four years and advanced dementia for two years. They had been married sixty years, and Elaine was now almost completely dependent on Ralph. She was also increasingly unpredictable. The week before, Ralph had found her in the kitchen, for some reason boiling water in several pots at once. Ralph had considered moving her to a nursing residence, but he hadn't found the time to look for one that might be suitable. He couldn't take her with him to look at these places, as she'd get too confused and anxious. Anyway, even if he did find one, he couldn't see how he could just dump her there and leave.

"I can't leave her alone for a minute," he would later tell his two adult children, Bill and Leslie.

"Dad, you should really let us help."

"No, I can handle this."

"But how? How can you take care of the house, make your phone calls, and always keep an eye on her?"

Ralph acknowledged it was difficult. But it was hard for him to ask for help.

Elaine had stayed at home, looking after the kids, and later in life belonged to several ladies' auxiliary organizations—clubs for "old ladies," she called them. Of course, now that she was so mentally impaired, she no longer participated. Ralph was a retired stockbroker; he was used to being in control. He had his hobbies—binding books by hand, a bit of golf, a touch too much alcohol (still much enjoyed)—and he had joined an Alzheimer's support group a few years back. He had not been there in a while.

Ralph had used several home cleaning services that his kids had arranged, but had since terminated them. "They tried to cheat me out of money," he said. "I can do a better job myself!"

Elaine's situation became much worse over the summer and fall of 2003. "We knew something of this," their son, Bill, later told the health professionals who were looking after Ralph. "We had no idea just how bad things were with our mom. Our dad never let on."

In March 2004, Ralph confided in Dr. Glass, his family doctor, that he would sometimes find Elaine in the living room or dining room with diarrhea running down her legs onto the floor. The smell would be just terrible. He would have to get her upstairs and settle her with a sedative, which, "thank goodness," he said, Dr. Glass had prescribed for her. He couldn't clean up with her awake. It would take hours to do so. Dr. Glass was worried about the toll this was taking on Ralph. Home care was arranged, two hours per week, with the intention to arrange for more.

Ralph insisted to Dr. Glass that despite the stress he was under, he was not depressed. He conceded that he was tired, that he didn't sleep as well as he used to, but thought that was to be expected. The family physician suggested Ralph see a colleague of his, a general internist with an interest in the mind-body connection. Bill went with his father to see Dr. Lo that same month. After examining Ralph thoroughly, Dr. Lo was reassuring. Ralph was as fit as a fiddle. He then made some recommendations. Ralph needed to get more exercise, walk more. Enjoy the fresh air and sunshine. Maybe try transcendental meditation.

"Dad laughed at that advice," Bill told me. "I was a bit surprised by those recommendations myself. Seemed like common sense to me."

The internist had told Ralph to avoid anti-anxiety pills because they could cause seizures, and to never take anti-depressants, because older people could get habituated to them and they could cause dementia. Dr. Lo also told him that if he wanted anti-depressants he could see a psychiatrist, but that he himself wouldn't prescribe them. Ralph had agreed with Dr. Lo.

"I can get better on my own," Ralph had told his kids, "so why take medication? I certainly don't have any hankering to see a shrink!" That seemed to be that.

No doubt Ralph knew that his wife would never improve. Dr. Glass recommended he consider "placing her" in a nursing home. Ralph found the idea of "placing" people offensive. "You place *things*, not people," he told his kids.

"I couldn't live with myself if I 'placed her,'" he told Dr. Glass. "Those homes are terrible places, not fit for human habitation." If Elaine went into a nursing home, Ralph would go with her. But he had no intention of doing any such thing, and he did not want to live by himself. So Ralph couldn't live with Elaine and he couldn't live without her.

"It wasn't just that week that was bad, it was his whole life," his children would later say. Perhaps he couldn't see any hope for the future. He must have been desperately unhappy. In late April 2004, Ralph did what no one could have ever imagined he would do.

Paul White, a neighbour who knew a little of Ralph's issues with Elaine, was out watering his lawn when he heard the shot. He just stood there for a moment, then put down his hose, walked quickly across the wet lawn, and knocked on Ralph's door. Getting no response, he let himself in using a key Ralph had given him. "Just in case, you know, should something happen to me . . . ," Ralph had told him. "You could maybe check on Elaine."

Paul called out but got no answer. He explored the house. Elaine was sleeping deeply upstairs. Nothing could have prepared Paul for what he found in the basement: Ralph in a large pool of blood, with half his face blown away, a discharged gun at his feet. Ralph had kept a loaded rifle in the basement. Maybe he was cleaning the rifle. Maybe it was attempted suicide. We will never know for sure.

Paul fumbled for his phone and desperately called 911.

Ralph was unconscious, still alive, barely. The police and emergency medical team arrived within minutes and intubated him at the scene to protect his airway. He was taken to the ER, where more definitive resuscitation measures were undertaken. Large-bore intravenous lines were inserted so blood products could be administered. He was sedated so he wouldn't struggle, and given narcotics for pain relief. The gaping gunshot wound in his cheek was cleaned and packed.

Ralph was soon transferred to the ICU. There he was more comprehensively assessed. His cardiovascular system and neurological system seemed intact. The gunshot had missed his brain. After a few days, the ICU staff thought his sedation might be lightened.

In the meantime, there was a decision to be made about Ralph's facial wound. It would be best to close it soon, although it would require some serious and prolonged plastic surgery. It wasn't an emergency situation; Ralph wasn't unstable, he wasn't obviously suffering, his bleeding had been stopped, and his breathing needed only a little assistance from a ventilator. Consent for the surgery was sought from his adult children.

Much to the surprise of the ICU team, Ralph's children declined to consent to the surgery.

The attending physician and the ICU team called an urgent family meeting—the first of many, it would turn out. I was called in as an ethics consultant. My role was to clarify the issues, to help the family and staff work towards a reasonable decision, and to try to help ensure all the right questions were posed and answered. As an ethicist, I could make notes, see the family, write in the chart, but the decisions made would be the responsibility of the attending physician—any recommendations I made could be ignored.

I was sitting in the Quiet Room with the ICU team (Ralph's nurse, the intensivist on duty, two residents, and a respiratory technician), the plastic surgeon, and Ralph's children.

Specializing in treating critically ill patients, the intensivist began. "Your dad has a terrible injury—probably self-inflicted, probably survivable. Please help us understand your views. Why won't you let the surgeon fix his wound?"

Bill cleared his throat. "Dad must have had good reasons to have done this. He was likely fed up with looking after our mother twenty-four hours a day. Who wouldn't be? My sister and I have discussed this and feel it would be best if you stop his treatment and just let him go."

His sister, Leslie, nodded. "That's right. We want you to stop everything."

"What troubles us," said one of the residents, "is that we don't understand what drove your father to do what he did at this time. From what you've told me, it seems so out of character for your father."

Neither Bill nor Leslie answered. I could sense that they, too, were a little baffled by their father's actions—how could he have done what he did with Elaine upstairs and having made no arrangements for her? It just didn't jibe with what everyone knew of Ralph. All the same, Ralph's children were insistent on stopping all his treatment.

The intensivist was clearly annoyed. He looked up from his laptop computer. "Are you *sure* about that? If we lighten his sedation, he may simply breathe on his own. Ralph is really not on life support. Yes, he's on a ventilator, but this is because we've snowed him under with so much analgesics and sedatives, we have to protect his ability to breathe." He explained that Ralph would wake up with a large hole in his face. "You understand the consequences of that, don't you? If he was depressed before, he will certainly be even more depressed on waking badly injured." Stopping everything at this time, he said, would certainly increase Ralph's suffering.

"What are the chances that, when he wakes up, he won't have lost any of his marbles?" Bill and Leslie asked.

"We're pretty sure that neurologically he is okay. The bullet didn't even graze his brain."

The risks and likely benefits of the proposed surgery were discussed. We also talked about the role of substitute decision makers and the importance of acting in a patient's best interests. It must have been pretty clear to Bill and Leslie that the team thought Ralph should have the facial surgery. Slipping from the neutral role I was meant to play, I agreed.

Leslie and Bill conferred quietly for a few minutes. Then Bill said, "We guess you're right." There was a reluctant tone in his voice. "Go ahead with the surgery." Whether they actually agreed with the decision or were a bit intimidated by the ICU gang is hard to say. The team members were relieved, as was I.

The operation took six hours, but it was a success. At least, the plastic surgeon was pleased with the result. Two days after the surgery, with Ralph still sedated and on the ventilator, a feeding tube was passed down his esophagus to his upper, or small, intestine. Unfortunately, the tube punctured a hole through his intestine, causing acidic intestinal fluids to leak into his abdominal cavity. The acid and bacteria began to eat away at Ralph's nearby organs. If he was treated promptly—with antibiotics and more surgery—his chances of recovery would be very high. Delayed or no intervention, especially in the elderly, results in a very elevated mortality rate. No one Ralph's age could survive without surgery.

Ralph's children drew a line in the sand: no more surgery.

"We never should have agreed to the first surgery!" they said. They were at their father's bedside, talking to his nurse. "He's eighty-six years old and a real trooper. But this is something else altogether."

The ICU team called for a surgical consultation. More family and team meetings were held.

The surgeon said in his consult note that it would be relatively easy to fix the intestinal injury—"an hour in the OR," simply wash out the peritoneal cavity, make sure there were no injured organs, and sew up the puncture wound. Without this intervention, Ralph would die in days. The surgeon claimed he would not be able to operate without the consent of Ralph's children, with whom he had discussed Ralph's situation.

I met with the surgeons and the rest of the team. "Ralph's kids may be well intentioned," I said, "but they aren't acting as substitute decision makers should." They were supposed to act in their father's best interests.

The surgeon remained unmoved. "They are *his* decision makers," he said, as if their decisions could not be challenged.

The team argued amongst themselves. Someone suggested that because Ralph's injury was "doctor-caused," it must be fixed irrespective of the children's wishes. Others agreed, saying that this was an emergency and as such the injury could be repaired without consent. The plastic surgeon, who had spent so much effort correcting the facial wound, was particularly irate about the other surgeon's refusal to operate. "Fixing that perforation is a minor operation!"

I asked the surgeon who was refusing to operate, "Wouldn't you want it fixed if it were *your* father in the bed?"

"No, I'm not sure I would."

"Pfft!" the plastic surgeon blurted out. He threw up his arms and stormed out of the ICU. My role as an ethicist had been to promote dialogue. I hadn't done so well.

A second surgeon was called in, but he, too, declined to operate. It was clear by now that, without a surgeon to operate, Ralph would die. The intensivist sat down again with Bill and Leslie and tried to better understand them and their perspective. What was their relationship like with their parents? Did they appreciate the possibilities for future care of their parents? At the end of this discussion, the intensivist was confident that Ralph's children were motivated by what they thought was best for him. But was this what Ralph really would have wanted?

Good medical care sees patients, family members, and the caring professionals as engaged in a joint process of identifying the shared goals of care—a mutual-benefit scenario whereby responsibilities are reinforced, goals and principles of treatment agreed upon in advance, and the burdens of decision making shared.

But what could have been the shared goals in *this* scenario? From the perspective of Ralph's children, the goal of care was to prevent their father from suffering further. From the intensivist's perspective, treating the case as an attempted suicide, the goal was to prevent irreversible harm and death. For the surgeons, the goal may have been to avoid making one bad outcome worse with more, and ultimately futile, treatment.

Is it possible to bring these varying perspectives together? Perhaps. But only through knowing the patient and his situation better. Why had he acted as he did?

Ralph had been suffering under the weight of caring for his wife. His children may not have realized how depressed he was—they did now, but seemed not to be aware of the wider options for care. Suicidal depression in the elderly is not uncommon, and it is just as treatable as it is in younger patients. If greater efforts had been made to overcome Ralph's skepticism about psychiatry and psychiatric drugs, could he have been persuaded to accept medication? Ralph clearly could have used better social supports as well. He appeared to be bearing the whole weight of the world on his shoulders.

In Ralph's case, empathy could go both ways—his children imagined how Ralph must have suffered before shooting himself; the medical team perceived Ralph's actions as a cry for help, not as a wish for no assistance. Ralph seemed to act impulsively and uncharacteristically in leaving his wife behind. The health care practitioners thus saw good reason to try to stand between Ralph and death. The two surgeons' reluctance to intervene seemed to stem more from pessimism, a feeling that further surgery at this point would be following the patient down a deep, dark hole. *If I were in his shoes, I'd want to be dead, too.*

The challenge for all involved in Ralph's care should have been to ward off this pessimism and convince his children that empathizing with Ralph did not necessarily mean letting him go. There might have been more than a slim possibility that Ralph, as with most suicidal patients who are rescued, would be happy, or at least relieved, to be alive and would not attempt suicide a second time. Geriatric psychiatry could have been involved, and his social isolation could have been addressed. This would have been a compassionate response to a self-inflicted injury.

Ralph's children did, however, know him better than any of those looking after him. They were sure that their father would not thank them for keeping him alive. The intensivist tried, one last time, to persuade his children to allow the surgery to go ahead. They remained firm. Ralph died two days later, never recovering consciousness.

I did not know Ralph or his wife before his arrival at the ICU (nor did anyone else at the hospital), but this was a hard outcome for me to accept. There were alternatives for care that were not explored. The possibilities of effective psychiatric care to alleviate his dark mood were not considered, for example. The intestinal surgery was minor compared to what he had already survived. In the end, Ralph was not offered the benefit of good medicine. The elderly are sometimes denied the best care just because they are old. By comparison, no matter how vigorously a family objected, health care professionals would never agree to withdrawing treatment from a younger patient who had apparently attempted suicide, unless such treatment is truly futile, without good reason.

There was no good reason—it was simply too soon—to let Ralph go.

IX

DEATH AND THE DOCTOR

For the second time that month, Mark was requesting a prescription for barbiturates from his family doctor, Dr. Maurice Genereux.[1] Mark had tested positive for HIV in 1988. Dr. Genereux had been his primary care doctor since then.

It was summer of 1995, and there were still few effective drugs with which to treat AIDS. Everywhere patients were dying of AIDS-associated malignancies and infections. Mark told his doctor that he had lost the last prescription for the sleeping pills and needed another.

Dr. Genereux wrote out a prescription for fifty tablets of Seconal, each containing 100 milligrams of secobarbital. "Remember, only one at a time at night," he said, barely looking up from his prescription pad. He didn't seem particularly worried about the prescription. When taken as directed and used for a short time, Seconal is a very good sedative and widely used. However, it is well known that when taken for longer periods, barbiturates become addictive, and more than ten pills taken at once can impair the patient's ability to breathe. Dr. Genereux would admit later that he knew Mark was not going to use the Seconal in the prescribed way; he was going to use the tablets to kill himself when he felt his HIV condition was too much to bear. Dr. Genereux had prescribed enough Seconal to kill a moose.

At the time, Mark was in a relationship with another HIV-positive patient. In early 1993, Mark had found a bottle of Seconal prescribed to his partner by Dr. Genereux. He pleaded with the doctor not to help his partner commit suicide. Dr. Genereux declined to discuss it, citing patient confidentiality. Mark's partner died of AIDS a few months later. Mark became despondent and had difficulty sleeping. He became obsessed with the idea that he, too, might develop AIDS and was determined to commit suicide if that happened.

Mark's fears were common at the time. Many saw an HIV-positive diagnosis as a death sentence. Some patients were so terrified of HIV and AIDS that they refused all treatment, fearing it might make them sicker (which it sometimes did). And some young men, like Mark, worried about a future downward spiral of health, and wanted to take pre-emptive action to prevent that from happening.

Mark would say later that he thought Dr. Genereux knew very well what he would use the Seconal for, and yet had complied with the request—neither taking the time to examine Mark nor inquiring about his intended use of the drug. "He knew I was contemplating suicide," Mark would say at trial. "He just didn't seem that interested." Later that same day, a friend of Mark's found him unconscious. Mark had ingested the entire bottle of Seconal. His friend saved his life by acting quickly and calling 911.

Mark blames only himself for his actions that day. He was at a low point in his life and acted impulsively. But he would say at trial that Dr. Genereux was like a "Pez dispenser of pills"—give him a list of the pills you wanted and he would prescribe them, no questions asked. It was this slap-dash attitude to prescribing lethal drugs that would get the doctor into so much trouble.

Mark was not the only patient asking Dr. Genereux for prescriptions for large doses of barbiturates. Arron had tested positive for HIV in 1989. He and his best friend, Robert, had been Dr. Genereux's patients since 1990. Arron hadn't had an AIDS-defining condition—no fungal pneumonia, no viral-induced skin cancers or retinitis—but he, too, was concerned he might develop AIDS.

Arron had a long history of licit and illicit drug use. He was also prone to depression and to violent outbursts. In August 1995, he asked for, and received from

Dr. Genereux, a quantity of Seconal, a prescription that was repeated a week later when, accompanied by Robert, he told the doctor he had lost the first prescription. Afterwards, at home, he told Robert that he now had enough Seconal to kill himself. He instructed Robert not to interfere if he used them. Arron never returned to Dr. Genereux.

The following April, nine months after filling the Seconal prescriptions, Arron took all the tablets at once. He told Robert that he didn't want to suffer with AIDS; he "wanted to die with dignity." When Arron lapsed into unconsciousness, Robert got frightened and called Dr. Genereux, telling him that Arron had ingested all the Seconal and asking whether he should call 911. Dr. Genereux instructed Robert to do nothing, that he knew why Arron had taken the pills, that Arron wanted to die. He arranged to come to the house the next morning to pronounce Arron dead. He listed the cause of death on the death certificate as "AIDS pneumonia."

Concerns were raised after Arron's death by the coroner's office. The regulatory college for doctors in Ontario and the Attorney General's office were notified. Dr. Genereux was subsequently charged with assisting at suicide and falsely testifying as to the cause of death on a death certificate.

Many of Dr. Genereux's patients considered him to be a friendly, concerned, and sympathetic—perhaps too sympathetic—physician. But he was also a troubled man.

He had a hard time resisting the entreaties of his patients and found it difficult to separate his own needs from those of his patients.

In 1971 Dr. Genereux had graduated from medical school in Alberta, but he failed his fellowship examinations. He went to live in Africa where, according to evidence at his trial, he became an alcoholic. He returned to Canada and worked in various remote locations as a family doctor for several years. His hospital privileges in an Alberta hospital were withdrawn when he was outed as being gay. Later he had to leave an Arctic hospital when it was discovered that he was addicted to drugs.

Then, for ten years, Dr. Genereux seemed to be reformed: he abstained from drugs, and he worked as a substance abuse counsellor in Toronto from 1984 to 1987. He opened his Toronto practice in 1987, largely serving patients with HIV and the gay male population.

In 1994, Dr. Genereux pleaded guilty before the Discipline Committee of the College of Physicians and Surgeons of Ontario to sexual offences involving six male patients. His licence was suspended for two years, but he was out of practice for only fifteen months, having satisfied his college-imposed conditions. In February 1995 his licence to practice was reinstated. Just five months later, he prescribed lethal doses of Seconal to Mark and Arron.

At his trial, Dr. Genereux pleaded guilty to two charges of aiding and abetting patients to commit suicide. In 1998, the college's Discipline Committee again

revoked his licence to practice medicine. In 1999 the
Court of Appeals for Ontario upheld Dr. Genereux's
sentence of two years less one day in jail for assisting suicide. He has the dubious honour of being the only doctor
in North America to be found guilty of, and imprisoned
for, this offence.

Dr. Genereux's patients, Mark and Arron, were not
terminally ill. They were not afflicted by the terrible
infections and malignancies that characterized patients
with advanced HIV. Though few in number, there were
drugs that could be used to ward off AIDS and to bolster the patient's immune system. Scores of clinical trials
were under way for promising anti-HIV medications.
Counselling and psychiatric support services that were
not explored for Mark or Arron had been helpful for
many other HIV-positive patients.

Dr. Genereux's actions were not the actions of a
trusted advocate for his patients. There was nothing
dignified about the choices he made, given the circumstances of his patients. His actions showed a profound
lack of respect for his patients. Dr. Genereux failed to
take due care—to understand his patients' circumstances
and *why* they felt so desperate that they would request a
lethal dose of medication.

And yet the doctor was not without his defenders.
At his trial his actions were defended by expert witnesses
who claimed that what he had done reflected a modern

rejection of the old-fashioned Hippocratic oath that prohibits a physician from assisting a patient intending to commit suicide. Modern physicians, it was argued, do not take the oath and so are not bound by its prohibitions. They went on to argue that the principle of autonomy suggests it is pure paternalism to put limits on the requests of competent, ailing patients. The court rejected this argument. Doctors, it said, had a professional duty to scrutinize requests for any drugs, but for lethal ones especially.

Witnesses for the defence also warned that sanctioning Dr. Genereux would send a chill through the community of palliative care and HIV-expert physicians. They feared that, when providing end-of-life care, if they even raised the topic of assisted suicide with their patients, they, too, might face criminal charges.

Against this, witnesses for the prosecution argued that, while there may be legitimate circumstances for complying with a patient's request to help them die, Arron's case did not fall into that category. He was far from critically ill and would not meet any test for being terminally ill. As I testified, Dr. Genereux's actions were akin to handing a loaded gun to an acutely suicidal patient.

But no evidence was offered to suggest that punishing Dr. Genereux would send a chill through the community of doctors looking after dying patients and those who were HIV-positive. The argument assumed that health care professionals could not distinguish between legitimate and illegitimate requests for palliation and aid in dying, between assisted dying and assisted suicide.

Most patients who want help in dying are not suicidal. They do not seek death so much as a way out of their suffering. If there were any other options, most would no doubt take them. The classic case used to bolster support for aid in dying is that of the driver stuck in a burning wreck: unable to be extricated, should he be helped to die quickly, or should he be forced to endure a torturous death? Would assistance at death in such circumstances not be appropriate—an act of mercy? The question is this: If you are soon going to die a horrible death, is a chosen, palliated death not a preferable option?

There are still those who would never assist at death—even that of someone trapped in a burning wreck. They would never stop their rescue efforts. They would continue to hope for a miraculous last-moment release. Whereas some might see such efforts as heroic, others would see them as hubris—we cannot save everyone. In some desperate cases, we should let the patient go, forgo rescue in favour of compassion. However, letting go becomes morally contentious when the patient is not close to death or has alternatives for care and survival.

Where there *is* agreement is over the stopping of care—in Canada and most other developed nations, capable patients have a well-recognized judicial right to refuse any and all care, life sustaining or otherwise.

Susan Wolf is a whip-smart lawyer who has served on presidential commissions on ethics and is a member of the prestigious Hastings Center in New York State, a private think tank on bioethics. For years she had been a well-known opponent of physician aid in dying, or PAD.[2] Then she had the experience of her own father's final illness. He, too, was a lawyer and had a very close bond with his daughter. When he was well and thriving, he had told her that if he ever became ill, even if he were in a persistent vegetative state, he would want "everything" done: "More deeply, he argued that the Holocaust was incompatible with the existence of God. There is no afterlife, he claimed. This is it, and he wanted every bit of 'it' on any terms."[3]

In 2002, he was diagnosed with head and neck cancer. At first his view was predictable: he wanted his caregivers to "spare no effort." By 2007, the reality of his illness had shifted his perspective. Despite every form of medical treatment, the cancer had spread. He was seventy-nine years old and had metastases to his liver and lungs. Increasingly weak and disheartened, he said that he wanted to stop "everything." Immobility and a clouded sensorium soon set in and he was, Wolf writes, "reduced to fearful dependence." Burdened by a massive bleed requiring multiple transfusions, he asked his daughter to "accelerate" his dying.

Her reflexive answer, in keeping with her opposition to PAD, was to deny her father's request. Nevertheless, she did, she says, seriously consider helping him die. She was comfortable with stopping his feeding tube and IV, but she was not prepared to hasten his death in any way. Her father died of his illness before any hard questions had to be answered.

Ms. Wolf is lucky that life or nature imposed itself on her father. She didn't have to face the hard questions that would have compelled her to make difficult choices. Life is not always so considerate. Patients can die in ways that are difficult to palliate—with "fearful dependence" that does not get resolved so rapidly. Still others have no terminal illness but linger on for years in the twilight existence of minimally conscious or vegetative states.

It was precisely because of a fear of lingering in a state of irremediable suffering that Gloria Taylor and Lee Carter (on behalf of her mother, Kay) decided to challenge Canada's constitutional prohibition on physician-assisted death in 2010. Kay Carter suffered from immobility and chronic pain due to severe spinal stenosis, a condition that results in the progressive compression of the spinal cord. Kay informed her family that she did not wish to live out her life as an "ironing board," lying flat in bed. Gloria had ALS, also known as Lou Gehrig's disease. They both feared an eventual state of dependence on others. Given their circumstances, they wanted to decide when and how they would die. On the one hand, if they could not look to others for assistance in dying, they might have to end their lives prematurely.

On the other hand, if they waited too long, they would be unable to help themselves to die and then would require the unlawful assistance of others to do so. This situation, they argued, contravened their constitutional rights. They would be forced either to terminate their lives prematurely, while they still were able to help themselves, or to wait and seek assistance at death in a "dark alley" at home or by strangers in a foreign land. (In early 2010, Kay asked her daughter Lee and Lee's husband, Hollis Johnson, to support and assist her in arranging an assisted suicide in Switzerland. They travelled with her for that purpose, and she died in a clinic there. Gloria died of sepsis, unrelated to ALS, in 2012, not long after the court's ruling. Before her death, Gloria had the satisfaction of knowing she was the first and only person in Canada to obtain a "constitutional exemption" from federal criminal code prosecution for assistance at suicide.)

In an extensively written decision, the B.C. Supreme Court ruled in favour of Gloria and Lee in 2012. Besides granting a constitutional exemption to Gloria, the court gave the federal government one year to change the law. This decision went against the 1993 decision of the Supreme Court of Canada in the case of Sue Rodriguez, also a B.C. patient with ALS. In the Rodriguez case the Supreme Court ruled against the right to assistance at death. The judges acknowledged that in denying Rodriguez's appeal, they were condemning her to suffer. But were they to grant her a right to assistance at suicide, they argued, they would open the floodgates to the murder of vulnerable, disabled patients. (There was little evidence for such a fear then and there is little evidence for it now.)

In one unexpected fell swoop, the B.C. court overturned Canadian legal orthodoxy and challenged medical orthodoxy almost everywhere as well. The attorney general of Canada appealed the ruling, and the B.C. Court of Appeal overturned the B.C. Supreme Court's decision, arguing that in accordance with an ancient and conservative legal rule of *stare decisis*—"stand by things decided"—lower courts should always follow the rulings of higher ones.

An appeal of *this* decision was made to the Supreme Court of Canada. In a unanimous decision, the court ruled that it was the Court of Appeal that had got it wrong: a lower court *could* overrule a higher court's ruling if the factual circumstances or the applicable law had changed. And this was precisely what the Supreme Court found. The factual circumstances *had* changed: as survey after survey has shown, a majority (now over 80 per cent) of the Canadian population is consistently in favour of some form of assisted death. Contributing to the decision as well was the changing legal environment: regulations had been devised in other jurisdictions that could protect the vulnerable from unwanted assistance at death.

This is a landmark ruling in Canada. It joins a host of other judicial rulings that have challenged and changed how medicine is practised in the country, such as *Reibl v.*

Hughes, which set new standards for informed consent; *R. v. Morgentaler,* which struck down the old abortion law that impinged on a woman's right to choose; and *Nancy B. v. Hôtel-Dieu de Québec* and *Malette v. Shulman,* which finally established the right of competent adults to refuse life-sustaining care.

As Canada has moved forward in the debate over physician-assisted death, public evidence given by patients with terrible diseases has contributed in vital ways to the overwhelming support among Canadians for some form of assisted dying. One of the most powerful voices was Dr. Donald Low's. Dr. Low was a well-respected microbiologist in Toronto. Diagnosed with a brain stem tumour in early 2013, he died in September of that year. A week before he died, he made a video advocating for the option of assisted suicide. The video is unsparing and brave. Dr. Low was not afraid to die, he said, but he was afraid of a prolonged and agonizing death: "I'm just frustrated not being able to have control of my own life, not being able to make the decision for myself when enough is enough." Palliative care was important, he said, but it could only do so much. It could not, for example, give him back his strength or restore his breathing. He was confident that opponents of his position would change their minds if they could they live in his body for twenty-four hours.

Dr. Low, in the end, died of his rapidly progressive disease and did not need to seek an earlier release. This is not an unusual outcome for many patients seeking an assisted death—they die of their disease or from other illnesses before requiring assistance with death. For at least some of these patients, knowing that option is available to them is itself a source of comfort and relief.

In the *Carter v. Canada* decision of 2015, the Supreme Court outlined circumstances that justify assistance at death for a competent adult who "(1) clearly consents to the termination of life and (2) has a grievous and irremediable medical condition (including an illness, disease or disability) that causes enduring suffering that is intolerable to the individual."[4]

These conditions are not very restrictive. It is interesting, for example, that nowhere does the decision say the person must have a terminal or even a physical illness. It also does not state that the patient must have exhausted all therapeutic options, although it's pretty clear that the court had in mind very ill patients—those, say, with advanced ALS or in the later stages of cancer. But the court allowed that physician-assisted suicide would be acceptable even in the case of osteoarthritis if the patient were immobile and in constant pain, as was the case for Kay Carter. (The decision notes that Kay "had extremely limited mobility and suffered from chronic pain." This is a condition common to many people.) Still, in the view of the court, "a properly administered regulatory regime is capable of protecting the vulnerable from abuse or error."

Some patients take a pre-emptive approach to their own deaths—dying on their own time, while reasonably well. They may have a terminal illness but not yet be terminally ill. Nagui Morcos was just such a patient. He was in his mid-fifties when he died in Toronto by his own hand in 2012 before he could be severely affected by the Huntington's disease gene he had inherited from his father. I do not know how he died—the media reported only that he did not die alone. His neurologist knew of his desire to die—as did his family—and found him rational and thoughtful. Nagui had watched his father die in pain, psychotic and unable to care for himself. He knew he was going to die and did not want to go that way. His wish for assistance at dying was a considered and "rational" one, one he explained in a letter, read at his memorial and later published in the *Toronto Star*.[5]

The idea of having a rational wish to die confounds doctors. We are taught to see all such wishes to end one's life as suicidal and as the product of depression or other psychiatric illnesses causing mental instability. Such states, if acute and likely to be acted upon, may call for restraints and a mandatory psychiatric evaluation. This response assumes that self-induced harms are always to be avoided and that attempts to end one's own life are always pathological.

But experience has shown otherwise. Death is not always the worst outcome. Nagui could see where his illness would take him. He took pre-emptive action even though to some his symptoms did not seem so bad: increased urinary frequency, insomnia, forgetfulness, falls, slurred speech. But Nagui knew these symptoms were warnings of what was to come. He could sense that his future life would crush his present one. He wanted to let go *before* the worst happened.

The American patient Brittany Maynard had a similar attitude. In a much-publicized story, she died just before her thirtieth birthday in the fall of 2014 after taking a lethal, but legally prescribed, dose of drugs in Oregon. She had moved there from California because Oregon allowed physician-assisted death. Brittany had been diagnosed with an incurable brain cancer less than a year before. She had undergone surgery, but the cancer returned, worse than ever, as it usually does with her particular disease. There is no effective treatment, and patients soon learn what to expect: seizures, stroke-like events, loss of the use of body parts, cognitive impairment. Few patients survive more than a year.

Unlike many terminally ill patients, Brittany was young and vivacious. She wanted no part of this terrible disease. She chose to end her life when "enough was enough," and she did so with the support of her family.

In the cases of Brittany, Nagui, Donald, Gloria, and Kay, modern medicine has met its match. Even medicine at its best is not able to cure their illnesses: ALS, advanced brain tumours, Huntington's disease, even end-stage arthritis, are all terrible diseases that herald only decline and suffering for patients.

It doesn't matter how reasonable or understandable choosing death over life might be; it still presents a problem for health care professionals. It is easier to agree on paper that certain patients have the right to, and should be allowed to, choose death. But what if *you* were the patient's doctor? It is much more difficult to be the direct agent of another's death. To actually write a prescription for a lethal dose of medication, knowing full well what it will be used for, is very different to practitioners than unplugging a life-sustaining piece of equipment and allowing a patient to die as nature takes its course. This psychological hurdle will, in my view, make it difficult, if not impossible, for many health care professionals to participate in assisted death.

It is sometimes argued that assisting at dying shouldn't be the purview of physicians. It probably shouldn't be— at least not solely, anyway. Careful oversight of these acts is needed, and such oversight should be provided by a multidisciplinary group that would include medical professionals, regulatory authorities, lawyers, and ethicists. This would help to ensure that physician-assisted death never becomes routine.

As modern medicine advances towards improved treatment for illnesses that are currently irreversible, cause much suffering, and are invariably lethal, we may lessen the need and the demand for assistance at death. After all, it is the lack of alternatives to care and the limits of medicine that fuel many of the requests for assistance at death.

X

BEYOND THE BLACK BAG

Bill Masters had just finished watching the evening news when he heard the rattling of a garbage can. His curiosity piqued, he went out to investigate. As there hadn't been any house lights on or the garbage put out next door in months, he'd assumed his eighty-six-year-old neighbour, Sonja Baruch, had moved.

But she hadn't moved. It was Sonja making all the noise. She seemed out of breath as Bill approached her. When Bill commented on how long it had been since he'd seen her, Sonja explained, her voice faint and tremulous, that she had been in Europe attending her husband Jakob's art show. Jakob, Sonja said, was staying on a little longer. Bill's concern increased; Jakob had been dead for more than a decade.

Sonja and Jakob had moved next door to Bill thirty years earlier. Bill knew little about them, other than that they were childless, were originally from Poland, and had lived in Israel for a decade before coming to Canada. After ten years as neighbours, Sonja finally told Bill, with more than a hint of pride, that Jakob was an artist who had had successful exhibitions in Tel Aviv, Toronto, and Montreal. Another five years passed before Bill was invited to look at Jakob's paintings. They reminded him of the work of Marc Chagall, swimming with bright colours and flying people.

Bill was pulled back to the present as his eyes surveyed the garbage cans and litter in the driveway. Over Sonja's shoulder he caught a glimpse of a house in chaos, and the woman in front of him looked nothing like the Sonja he knew. She was unkempt: her hair uncombed, her fingernails uncut and coated with grime, her clothing stained and worn. She was no longer the dignified woman who had always carried herself like a queen, despite being barely four foot ten. She was too thin, malnourished almost. Sonja also looked scared, wide-eyed like a tiny deer caught in headlights.

Bill asked Sonja how she was managing without Jakob around. She admitted she was a bit behind on her housework but declined Bill's offer of assistance. Then, as she was retreating to her door, Sonja lost her balance and tumbled backwards, striking her head on the cement. She was bleeding profusely from a large scalp laceration.

Bill called 911. The firefighters, police, and finally the ambulance all arrived. It was obvious that Sonja was delirious. At first she balked and put up a little resistance to being treated, but then she relented. She was whisked off to the hospital, where she was diagnosed with dehydration and "failure to thrive."

Before Sonja was taken away, Bill had the foresight to ask her for a key so he could lock up her house or let someone in if Sonja should need anything. Bill would later admit to us that he couldn't resist looking inside the home, although he said he felt a little like a voyeur. Sonja's house was an unmitigated disaster. There was garbage everywhere. Rooms and hallways were piled floor to ceiling with old magazines, newspapers, and flyers. The kitchen sink, once porcelain white, was now blackened with dirt. Worst of all was her bathroom—a feces-filled toilet, and next to it a bucket encrusted with soiled toilet paper. Not only was there no electricity, there was no running water. Bill did not linger. The stench was too awful.

Sonja was admitted to a ward in my hospital, and during the second month of her stay I was called in by her nursing staff to act as an ethicist on her case. I was asked to assess her mental capacity to decide where she could live. Initially resistant to being admitted, Sonja now did not want to leave—at least not to go to the nursing home where the discharge planner wanted to send her. Sonja wanted to go home. Was that a viable option? If not, could she be "coerced" into a chronic care facility?

Sonja had been admitted *three previous times* that year: the first time for cellulitis, a serious skin infection in one of her legs; the second time for bacterial pneumonia; and the third time, just two months before her fall, for low blood sugar (likely, we later realized, the result of being in a starved state, having so little food in her home). On the last two admissions, Sonja was noted to be somewhat confused. She had two brain CAT scans, and although they didn't indicate any stroke or tumour, she did have "mild to moderate" atrophy. The confusion was considered transient and had cleared sufficiently after each admission that she had been released to go home.

Sonja's in-hospital care had been exemplary, and yet when I inspected her chart, I found no evidence that anyone had thought to consider how she would function back at home. Where was the occupational therapy assessment, for example? Where was the regional geriatric program that would follow vulnerable patients like Sonja into their homes? Maybe these services were swamped. Maybe Sonja's grace and regal carriage fooled her health care professionals into thinking she was not like "the others." I suspected, though, that even if some help had been offered, Sonja would have declined it. She did not trust strangers. Still, there was no record that anyone had even tried.

On this admission, however, once her dehydration and head injury were treated, Sonja's confusion came to the fore, and her cognitive impairment was taken more seriously. The proper assessments were done. She was not just transiently confused; she was diagnosed as being in a moderately advanced stage of dementia.

Sonja had no interest in being confined to a nursing home. To place her in a chronic care facility, we would have had to ignore her protests, and the almost certain knowledge that she would be desperately unhappy there. So we returned to the option she preferred. There was only one way to gauge the feasibility of her returning home—we had to go there. The hospitalist (a doctor with general medical training who looks after in-hospital patients) went himself, and I went along for the ride.

I have had patients who were hoarders, but their homes were clean as a whistle compared to Sonja's. As we toured her house, we discovered her water had been turned off six months earlier and her power two months before that. The food in her fridge was rotting; her cupboards were bare. No wonder Sonja kept getting ill. Her house must have been in this appalling state the last two times she had been released from the hospital and possibly the time before that as well. We met Bill and some of Sonja's other neighbours who, although aware of her vulnerability, had been unable to help her, as she resisted all offers of assistance and was a very private person.

Sonja obviously could not return to her home in its present state. She lacked insight into how bad the condition of her house was, and she was clearly having difficulty in managing her financial affairs. Hospitalization offered her a brief respite from her living conditions. She recognized that her mind wasn't as sharp as it used to be, and, as much as she wanted to be in her home, she was afraid to live alone. She was scared of rogue invaders and anxious about going out shopping on her own. However, while she could vaguely appreciate the dangers of returning home alone, and at times was fearful of it, nothing could dissuade her from the idea. Home was where she "belonged," she said.

In conversation with her, I learned that her small house represented her whole life: it was her refuge, a tribute to her late husband and the life they had shared for decades. It was understandable that she did not want to leave it behind. If the disrepair of her home was a reflection of her impaired cognition, was there a way we could address her medical condition while accommodating her fervent desire to live at home? Sonja had no family and she had not designated anyone to manage her estate or make medical decisions for her. As it turned out, however, unlike with many isolated patients, Sonja's financial resources were considerable. Had she not had the funds she had, the unfair and unfortunate truth is that she would have been institutionalized without her consent or assent. Instead, the hospitalist was able to make an astute decision. He stepped aside from his formal role as her "hospital doctor" and acted as her defender and her advocate: he asked the Public Guardian's office to release some of her funds to fix her house and he personally oversaw the cleanup. Sonja would stay in hospital for an extra month and would leave of her own accord once her house was ready. (The hospital's extension was possible in the 1990s, before today's 120 per cent occupancy that sees patients spilling into the hallways and byways. It is unlikely that Sonja's longer stay could now be accommodated.)

When Sonja was settled back in her home, I became her family doctor and made regular house calls to her. I was amazed to see her transformation. Bright, smiling from ear to ear, she was delighted to be on her own in her rejuvenated home. The kitchen sink was sparkling white, and her bathroom was immaculate once again. Her late husband's paintings hung proudly on newly painted walls. Most important, she could afford, for the next several years at least, round-the-clock live-in help. We could not cure Sonja's dementia, but we could help her live as she wanted. She could have her tea, her bread, and honey just the way she had always liked them. This meant everything to her. Sonja not only survived; she thrived.

Sonja did not have to return to hospital or the ER again. She died in her sleep at home two years later.

Sonja's care was not headline news. It did not require the use of any fancy technology. Of course Sonja benefited from CAT scans, rigorous blood work, and skilled nursing care, the best the system could offer, better than many individuals get. But she survived because a concerned neighbour looked in on her. And she thrived because one of her doctors went outside the walls of his institution to support her until she could safely go home.

Sonja's story suggested to me something important about health care. Good medicine is not just what is good *for* you; it is also what is seen and felt to be good *by* you. It takes into account and tries to accommodate your desires, wishes, fears, and beliefs. One measure of the success of medicine lies in stories like Sonja's—small victories, desires recognized and met, souls counselled and comforted, promises kept, and duties fulfilled.

Sometimes the success of care will require all the benefits that revolutionary advances in medical care can offer: the life-altering, life-saving potential of stem cells; the transformation of care made possible by the mapping of the human genome. It is possible not only to predict with unprecedented accuracy whether an individual will develop an illness now or many years into the future, but also whether an individual will respond positively to recommended treatments. Some diseases do remain too complex to be predicted in quite this way, and this type of care is still too expensive to be widely accessible. However, the potential to determine the true genomic uniqueness of each patient in such specific and purposeful ways will continue to revolutionize the nature of "personalized" medical care.

And yet we need to match our investment in such advances in knowledge and treatments with a commitment to the kind of personalized care that served Sonja so well. Sonja was able to escape the nursing-home trajectory of many failing, elderly patients only because she had the independent means to do so. It is the distressing reality that even in a country as rich as Canada, the best care, the most ethical care, that patients want and need is, because of limited resources and financial constraints, too often out of reach.

Whether we are considering the benefits of genomic medicine or palliative care, when it comes right down to it, what is ultimately best for a patient is almost always arrived at in conversation with their physicians. These critical conversations are not always easy to have. Often we wait too long—the patient becomes too ill, too advanced in their symptoms, too close to death to engage in more intimate discussions about what the future holds and what treatment alternatives there might be. In my own journey through the land of illness, I have often avoided these conversations myself. At times I was too ill; at other times the circumstances did not seem right. Sometimes I didn't want to face the illness before me or what I worried my future might bring. The hazard of being a patient who is also a doctor is that it is sometimes easier, though not always better for you, to try to arrange your own diagnosis and care. I postponed some hard decisions about my Parkinson's, and I found ways to avoid acknowledging that things were getting worse. I assumed I had done everything that could be done. I minimized the impact of Parkinson's on my life. I didn't discuss with my neurologist my disabled gait, my slow pace, my loss of balance. My strategy of evasion is a common one among people with a serious illness. It isn't so much that we are in denial as unable or unwilling to see our condition from the outside. From inside my illness it was easy to miss the extent to which I had adapted to my worsening symptoms. I was the proverbial frog in hot water, in ever-increasing danger of being boiled to death.

In the fall of 2013, I finally realized I had to do something. I was at an international conference on Parkinson's in Montreal and looking at the thousands of people in attendance, many of whom had Parkinson's, and I realized that my gait was among the worst there. Then, as I was resting on a bench, trying to summon the strength to cross the street, I had a moment of clarity: I could see my illness and myself from the outside. I did not want to spend the rest of my days in a wheelchair. My friends might be willing to push me around, but I wanted something more. On that bench in Montreal I considered the possibilities that had been offered and were open to me. Things could be worse, I recall thinking; I could have an illness that was not treatable. Mine was. *I will get better*, I thought to myself. I just had to make the right choice.

I returned to Toronto and called my neurologist. I had been a patient of her clinic for over a year. I had done physiotherapy and exercises, tried various walking aids and braces. I had had Botox injections to try to reduce the spasm in my left leg. In that time I had experienced no real improvement. After months of gentle persuasion, she was happy to hear I would now consider deep brain stimulation. She was reassuring, optimistic about how I would benefit from the procedure. And I did.

My fiercest hope in all of this was that I might be able to stop my decline, to preserve the functions I had and even, if possible, turn back the clock. To walk again unaided, if only for a limited time, was my goal. These are outcomes, simple ones, familiar to and hoped for by all patients: to re-experience an element of normalcy, whatever the dysfunction might be, for however long that element might last. It took me years to "come out" with my illness, and it was only once I had made the decision to have surgery that I could more honestly look at my life. My initial jubilation at the near disappearance of my Parkinsonian gait after my surgery has been replaced by a more measured, albeit still optimistic, approach to life. A door to a better life has been pried open. How long it will remain so is impossible for anyone to say.

Whether the recipients of the best designer cancer drugs or the most intricate forms of surgery, many patients like me still wait anxiously to see what their future holds. Once struck by and successfully treated for a serious cancer, no one ever feels completely out of the woods; most patients will always have some concern that the malignancy may recur. Successful transplant recipients never quite stop fearing that a donor's organ may one day be rejected. I continue to be followed by my neurologist and neurosurgeon. Whether and at what point anything more can be done for me will depend in part on the state of medical research. It will turn as well on my ability to acknowledge any further decline. I must remain vigilant, willing to accept ongoing care and medical surveillance. I'm not convinced that having a serious condition makes anyone, on his or her own, more insightful. We will always need caring practitioners who can see through our defences and denials, our deceptions and delusions. No matter how simple or complex our illnesses may be, the empathic connection between patients and physicians is the moral core of medical care. It is the art of good medicine.

NOTES ON SOURCES

INTRODUCTION: STRANGERS IN A STRANGE LAND

1. D. Neuhauser, "Oliver Wendell Holmes M.D. 1809–94 and the Logic of Medicine," *Quality and Safety in Health Care* 15, no. 4 (2006): 302, http://dx.doi.org/10.1136/qshc.2006.019398.
2. As quoted in A. Knoll, "The Reawakening of Complementary and Alternative Medicine at the Turn of the Twenty-First Century: Filling the Void in Conventional Biomedicine," *Journal of Contemporary Health Law and Policy* 20, no. 2 (2004): 349n157.

CHAPTER 1: BAD ATTITUDE

1. *Reibl v. Hughes*, [1980] 2 SCR 880, http://scc-csc.lexum.com/scc-csc/scc-csc/en/item/2563/index.do.
2. *Arndt v. Smith*, [1997] 2 SCR 539, http://scc-csc.lexum.com/scc-csc/scc-csc/en/item/1527/index.do.
3. G. Robertson, "Informed Consent 20 Years Later," *Health Law Journal Special Edition* (2003).

4. M. Sinclair, *The Report of the Manitoba Pediatric Cardiac Surgery Inquiry: An Inquiry into Twelve Deaths at the Manitoba Health Sciences Centre in 1994* (Manitoba: Provincial Court of Manitoba, 1995).

CHAPTER 3: THROWN FOR A LOOP

1. This was well documented by Oliver Sacks in his 1973 book, *Awakenings*.
2. G. R. Baker et al. "The Canadian Adverse Events Study: The Incidence of Adverse Events Among Hospital Patients in Canada," *CMAJ: Canadian Medical Association Journal* 170, no. 11 (2004): 1678–86.

CHAPTER 5: A DEATH FORETOLD, A DEATH UNFOLDS

1. I have used his real name, as I have done with the names of some of the doctors involved in these stories where they are relevant and in the public domain.

CHAPTER 6: THE QUALITY OF OUR MERCY

1. These are the real names of the patient and his family. Their consent to use their names and write this chapter was obtained.
2. *Cuthbertson v. Rasouli*, [2013] 3 SCR 341, http://scc-csc.lexum.com/scc-csc/scc-csc/en/item/13290/index.do.
3. S. Blackburn, *Mirror, Mirror: The Uses and Abuses of Self-Love* (Princeton: Princeton University Press, 2014), 16.

CHAPTER 7: SUFFER THE CHILDREN

1. This chapter is based entirely on documents in the public record (other than the story of Christine Ho, who was obviously my patient). I had no access to the health records of these patients.

2. The Six Nations is a confederacy of the six Iroquois nations in southern Ontario. The Mississaugas of the New Credit First Nation is nearby but is an Ojibwe nation.

3. *Gillick v. West Norfolk and Wisbech Area Health Authority*, [1986] 1 AC 112 (H.L.).

4. R. Wheeler, "Gillick or Fraser? A Plea for Consistency over Competence in Children: Gillick and Fraser Are Not Interchangeable," *BMJ: British Medical Journal* 332 (2006): 807.

5. See the Supreme Court of Canada's ruling in *A.C. v. Manitoba* that authorized giving a blood transfusion to a fourteen-year-old Jehovah's Witness: "The more serious the nature of the decision and the more severe its potential impact on life or health, the greater the degree of scrutiny required" (*A.C. v. Manitoba*, [2009] 2 SCR 181, http://scc-csc.lexum.com/scc-csc/scc-csc/en/item/7795/index.do).

6. Priscilla Alderson, personal communication to the author.

7. P. Alderson, *Children's Consent to Surgery* (Buckingham, U.K.: Open University Press, 1994), 3.

8. Nahnda Garlow, "CAS Closes Case on Ojibwe Child; 'We Respect Makayla's Choice,'" *Two Row Times*, May 20, 2014, http://www.tworowtimes.com/news/cas-closes-case-on-ojibwe-child-we-respect-makaylas-choice/.

9. Tom Blackwell, "Makayla Sault's Parents Say They Have No Regrets over Girl's Decision to Opt for Holistic Cancer Treatment," *National Post*, June 6, 2014, http://news.nationalpost.com/news/canada/makayla-saults-parents-say-they-have-no-regrets-over-girls-decision-to-opt-for-holistic-cancer-treatment.

10. See, for example, Connie Walker, "First Nations Family's Refusal of Chemo a Precedent-Setting Case, Expert Says," CBC News, October 16, 2014, http://www.cbc.ca/news/aboriginal/first-nations-family-s-refusal-of-chemo-a-precedent-setting-case-expert-says-1.2800883.

11. Jonathan Garlow, "Fighting On in Memory of Makayla Rain," *Two Row Times*, June 17, 2015, http://www.tworowtimes.com/new/ fighting-on-in-memory-of-makayla-rain.

12. *Minister of Social Services v. F. and L. Paulette* (1991), Saskatchewan Provincial Court, Sask. D. 1568-1605 (unreported).

13. Thanks to Ryan Giroux for this suggestion.

14. Gloria Galloway, "Ontario First Nations Girl Taken Off Chemotherapy Has Died," *The Globe and Mail*, January 19, 2015, http://www.theglobeandmail.com/life/health-and-fitness/health/ health-care-must-do-better-at-respecting-aboriginal-patients -journal-urges/article22517597/.

15. *Hamilton Health Sciences Corp. v. D.H.*, 2014 ONCJ 603, http:// canlii.ca/t/gf8sg.

16. Susan Gamble, "Best Interests of Child 'Paramount,'" *Brantford Expositor*, April 24, 2015, http://www.brantfordexpositor. ca/2015/04/24/best-interests-of-child-paramount.

17. L. Richardson and M. Stanbrook, "Caring for Aboriginal Patients Requires Trust and Respect, Not Courtrooms," *CMAJ: Canadian Medical Association Journal* 187, no. 3 (2015), http://dx.doi. org/10.1503/cmaj.141613.

CHAPTER 9: DEATH AND THE DOCTOR

1. The names in this chapter are not fictional, and the actions and words attributed to patients are entirely based upon information in documents such as court proceedings and newspaper articles. I gave evidence for the prosecution at Dr. Genereux's criminal trial.

2. S. Wolf, "Physician-Assisted Suicide," *Clinics in Geriatric Medicine* 21 (2005): 179–92.

3. S. Wolf, "Confronting Physician-Assisted Suicide and Euthanasia: My Father's Death," *The Hastings Center Report* 38 (Sept-Oct 2008): 23–26.

4. *Carter v. Canada*, [2015] 1 SCR 331, http://scc-csc.lexum.com/scc
-csc/scc-csc/en/item/14637/index.do.

5. "Huntington's Disease Sufferer Nagui Morcos Explains His
Suicide," *Toronto Star*, September 7, 2012, http://www.thestar.com/
news/gta/2012/09/07/huntingtons_disease_sufferer_nagui
_morcos_explains_his_suicide.html.

ACKNOWLEDGEMENTS

This book would not have been possible without the support, encouragement, and inordinate work of my editors, family, friends, and colleagues. Words of very special thanks go out to my ebullient and unsurpassable editor at Doubleday Canada, Martha Kanya-Forstner, who originally suggested this project, without whom it would not have happened, and who meticulously guided me along the way, tolerating my innumerable revisions right up to the very last moment. Many thanks must be made to Shaun Oakey, my careful copy editor. And special thanks to my very good friend Nancy Carroll of Wordreach, an editor extraordinaire who has encouraged my writing in many ways. Many thanks must also go to all the patients and families who appear in this book, disguised or not. I have tried to be fair to their stories. Much gratitude to Priscilla Alderson, my writing class at the University of Toronto under Shaughnessy Bishop-Stall, Wendell Block, Monica Branigan, Franco Carlevale, Kristine Connidis, Marla Feldman, Rob Fowler, Ryan Giroux, Samantha Haywood, Craig Hébert, Janice Hébert, Paul Hébert, Ann Heesters, Marlene Kadar, Hannah Kaufman, Michael Kaufman, Miriam Kaufman, Daniel Marrone, Maria McDonald, Cliodhna McMullin, Sandi Mulvihill, Brian Murray, Judy Rebick, Gordon Rubenfeld, Jacob Scheier, Laura Sky, Robert Storey, Polly Thompson, Suzanne Weiss, Shawn Winsor, Cassandra Wolfe, and b. h. Yael. Special thanks to my two children, Raven and Neil, for their helpful comments on several chapters. And, of course, final thanks must go to my wife, Victoria, my source of support and succour in all times good or bad, and who exercised the keenest of eye and ear in her edits of this book.

My deepest appreciation for all the aid in writing I have received. The errors and limitations of the text remain my own.